REBEL BODIES

A guide to the gender health gap revolution

SARAH GRAHAM

GREEN TREE
LONDON · OXFORD · NEW YORK · NEW DELHI · SYDNEY

GREEN TREE
Bloomsbury Publishing Plc
50 Bedford Square, London, WC1B 3DP, UK
29 Earlsfort Terrace, Dublin 2, Ireland

BLOOMSBURY, GREEN TREE and the Diana logo are trademarks of Bloomsbury
Publishing Plc

First published in Great Britain 2023

A catalogue record for this book is available from the British Library

Library of Congress Cataloguing-in-Publication data has been applied for add where a
UK originated single-ISBN edition for which we own US rights

ISBN: HB: 978-13994-0111-1; eBook: 978-13994-0109-8; ePdf: 97813994-0114-2

2 4 6 8 10 9 7 5 3 1

Typeset in Minion Pro by Deanta Global Publishing Services, Chennai, India
Printed and bound in Great Britain by CPI Group (UK) Ltd., Croydon, CR0 4YY

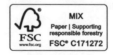

MIX
Paper | Supporting
responsible forestry
FSC® C171272

To find out more about our authors and books visit www.bloomsbury.com
and sign up for our newsletters

CONTENTS

The personal is political

1

'The personal is political': Introduction

When I first became a feminist, I was fascinated by the second-wave notion of consciousness-raising groups. Popularised by American feminists in the late 1960s and 1970s, these groups involved women sitting together, sharing their experiences and realising – often for the first time in their lives – that they weren't alone. Fifty years before #MeToo trended on Twitter, women were having their own 'me too!' realisations, and uniting over their shared experiences of sexism, discrimination and oppression.

I imagined them sitting around each other's living rooms, comparing notes over a cuppa or a G&T – or whatever the feminist tipple du jour was – about how, despite increasing rights in the workplace, they were still doing all the housework, childcare was unaffordable, and their husbands wouldn't even pick their socks up off the bathroom floor. How little has changed.

As my interest in health journalism grew, I also became fascinated by the gynae workshops of the second wave, where women armed with hand mirrors and specula sought to educate and empower one another to know their own bodies – or at the very least to take a look 'down there' for the first time in their lives. Germaine Greer famously encouraged women to taste their own menstrual blood, but far more significant and overlooked was the educational work of health activist organisations like the Boston Women's Health Book Collective, which produced the landmark women's health publication, *Our Bodies, Ourselves,* in the US.

It was this kind of vital consciousness-raising work that gave rise to my favourite feminist slogan: the personal is political. The title of a 1970 Carol Hanisch essay, 'the personal is political' highlights the intersection between personal experience and broader socio-political contexts. It is, in the words of Black feminist scholar Kimberlé Williams Crenshaw, 'The process of recognising as social and systemic what was formerly perceived as isolated and individual.'

Today, of course, much of what was once dismissed as merely the private, personal concerns of a few women has infiltrated the political and legal sphere. We have gender pay gap legislation, for example, maternity rights and the legal recognition (as recently as 1991) that non-consensual sex within marriage is rape. At the time of writing, 35% of British MPs are women and – on paper at least – we've never been better off.

But, despite those gains, so much of what was pissing off feminists in the 1960s is still pissing us off today. The personal is still very much political, and what could be more personal than health? Our mental and physical health impacts on every single aspect of our lives, cutting across work, family, relationships, culture and political engagement. Not only does our health impact on our ability to participate equally in society, but the decisions of political leaders – whether that's funding for research or cuts to public services – also impact on our everyday health and wellbeing.

The most obvious example is abortion, which remains the single most politicised healthcare procedure on the planet. With politicians apparently incapable of keeping their noses out of our uteruses, abortion is understandably the most prominent health issue for mainstream feminism and has been for quite some time. But feminist health activism doesn't begin and end with reproductive rights – although for many years I mistakenly believed it did.

As easy as it is to dismiss health as a personal, private matter, the politics of women's health have wide-reaching effects across the whole of society, impacting on patients' families, relationships and employers. From a purely financial perspective, endometriosis alone is estimated to cost the UK economy £8.2 billion a year, while 14 million working days per year are lost to the menopause. Yet these health issues, and many more, remain marginalised, under-researched and dismissed as 'normal' or unimportant by the medical profession. That attitude doesn't just hurt affected individuals and their families: the literal cost to society is huge.

The more time I've spent researching and writing about women's health, the more I've realised that gender bias cuts across the whole healthcare spectrum. Sexism – and all the other forms of discrimination with which it intersects – affects women's health, and the health of trans men, intersex and non-binary people, from our heads to our toes, from birth to death, all over the world. And these health inequalities can be fatal: women are up to three times more likely than men to die from a heart attack and Black women are four times more likely than white women to die in childbirth.

*

Many of these disparities are deeply rooted in historic attitudes and beliefs about women's bodies, bodies of colour, disabled bodies, queer, trans and intersex bodies – in fact, any bodies that don't fit the archetypal cisgender (not trans), white, able-bodied male 'norm' that medicine has long taken as its default model. These bodies are seen as 'other', dismissed as inherently unruly and disruptive, and have long been neglected, poorly understood, or else used and abused by medical science.

As early as 1900 BC, an Ancient Egyptian medical papyrus attributes women's 'behavioural disturbances' to their 'wandering wombs', which were believed to roam around the body causing mischief. This notion of what we now know as 'hysteria' (from

3

the Greek word *hystera*, meaning uterus) was popularised by Ancient Greek medical pioneer Hippocrates – whose name, thanks to the Hippocratic Oath, is still closely associated with the codes of medical ethics that doctors follow today.

The Greeks and other ancient civilisations held the troublesome uterus responsible for countless physical and mental symptoms. Hysteria was associated with such unwomanly conditions as failure to marry or bear children, as well as reproductive health issues like absent periods (amenorrhea), miscarriage and the menopause. Indeed, as feminist cultural historian Elinor Cleghorn writes in *Unwell Women*, 'Since their sole purpose was to bear and raise children, women's health was entirely defined by their uteruses.'

By the 19th century – after a lengthy period of being linked with witchcraft and satanic possession – hysteria had been reimagined, most famously by Sigmund Freud, as a psychological condition. Freud's *Studies on Hysteria* helped to establish the still-persistent association between hysteria and so-called 'conversion' or 'psychosomatic' disorders. His theories gave rise to the belief still seen today that if medicine can't otherwise explain a woman's symptoms, they must all be 'in her head', triggered by her own neuroses or by the repression of sexual trauma.

This diagnosis of hysteria, having been variously used to explain everything from period pain to wifely disobedience, was removed from the standard US clinical handbook, *Diagnostic and Statistical Manual of Mental Disorders*, just 40 years ago, in 1980. But the spectre of the ultimate 'female malady' still haunts surgeries and hospitals across the UK.

Hysteria, and the ideas associated with it, also feed into broader feminist issues. Its echoes are there when women are shut down for being 'too emotional' or 'hormonal', for 'over-reacting', being 'too demanding' or 'unladylike'. Women, in short, who don't know our place. We are not only defined by our bodies, but also constrained by them – too in thrall to the whims of our hormones to be trustworthy, rational or competent at anything other than

4

our natural, biological purpose. This attitude has been used to justify excluding women from positions of power for millennia. It's equally present when women are accused of 'crying rape', or when cis women and trans people are denied autonomy over their own bodies. The message is simple: we cannot be trusted.

All of this, of course, is before we even begin to explore the many intersecting biases and oppressions that contribute to so many patients' experiences. Like the rest of Western society, medicine has a long history of colonialism and racial bias, of legitimising homophobia and transphobia, of ableism, ageism, classism and more. These prejudices may simply reflect those of our broader society, but, when it comes to the medical profession, they can quite literally be a matter of life or death.

Most notably, in the context of women's health, the so-called 'Father of Modern Gynaecology', James Marion Sims, experimented on the bodies of Black, enslaved women in the US, without anaesthesia, on the basis that these women 'felt less pain'. This racist myth still haunts medical practice to this day, with Black patients 22% less likely than white patients to be prescribed pain medication and 29% less likely to be treated with opioids. A US study as recently as 2016 found that half of white medical students and postgraduate trainees held false beliefs about Black people, contributing to racial disparities in the assessment and treatment of pain.

*

This legacy of injustice and oppression has created a perfect storm for health inequalities to flourish. Understandably, it's also led to considerable mistrust of the healthcare profession among marginalised communities. But the tide is turning, slowly.

We're living through a fascinating era of activism and transformation, with vast cultural movements shifting the conversation on racism, trans rights, sexual violence, period poverty and more. When you scratch the surface of each of these issues – from #MeToo to #BlackLivesMatter – many of the same themes emerge: trust, dignity, compassion, equality, and the importance of hearing, acknowledging and believing people's accounts of their own experiences, trauma and pain.

At the same time, the Covid-19 pandemic has put health – in all its private, personal, public and political interconnectedness – firmly at the forefront of everyone's consciousness. Vital conversations about the social and political determinants of health are finally taking the spotlight, but activists and patient advocates have been laying the groundwork for years.

As a women's health journalist, I have spent much of my career so far talking to and being inspired by women – cis, trans, queer, straight, old, young, middle-aged, Black, white, Asian, fat, thin, disabled, non-disabled, working class, wealthy and everything in between – who have found themselves at the sharp end of both conscious and unconscious bias in healthcare.

I've heard countless stories of doctors dismissing women's pain, often with attitudes that seemed to be a hangover from the pre-feminist past. Worse still, many of these women had been disbelieved and invalidated into doubting their own experiences – a medical form of gaslighting that left them wondering if maybe it really was in their heads after all. Similar experiences are documented by Baroness Julia Cumberlege in her 2020 *First Do No Harm* report, which investigated the women's health scandals surrounding vaginal mesh implants and birth defects caused by both the Primodos pregnancy test and the epilepsy medicine sodium valproate. The report describes: 'a culture of dismissive and arrogant attitudes that only serve to intimidate and confuse… [and a] widespread and wholly unacceptable labelling of so many symptoms as "normal" and attributable to "women's problems".'

This isn't just the case for cis women. Trans and non-binary people navigating the healthcare system encounter strikingly similar attitudes – and worse. Writing for the *Guardian* in 2013, journalist Jane Fae asked, 'Has your doctor ever laughed in your face during an appointment? Denied that your condition exists?

Or simply told you that you're too ugly to merit treatment? Outrageous? Yes, but also pretty much par for the course if you happen to be trans.'

She details the 'world of abuse and humiliation' trans patients face when interacting with healthcare professionals, even in consultations about non-trans specific health issues. As for making a complaint, she adds, 'Few will risk it: most are cowed into silence by the tacit threat that rocking the boat could lead to a termination of their desperately needed treatment.'

It's an imbalance of power that has long been a barrier for the most marginalised of patients and highlights exactly why trans healthcare is every bit a feminist issue. If we care, as I do, about bodily autonomy, reproductive justice and equal access to healthcare, then the health of trans and non-binary people must absolutely be a part of the conversation.

*

In 2018 I met women's health activist Clare Knox for a cup of tea that quickly turned into cocktails. After a couple of hours putting the world to rights, I came away feeling more impassioned and fired up than ever – not just about the issues we'd been discussing, but also the importance of elevating women's voices and experiences. Inspired by our conversation, I founded Hysterical Women, a trans-inclusive feminist health blog that curates and explores stories of the dismissal, gaslighting and misdiagnosis that cis and trans women, and anyone assigned female at birth, experience when accessing healthcare.

The blog was, and still is, an effort to unpick the sexism behind women's healthcare experiences, as well as exploring the impact of racism, ageism, ableism, classism, homophobia, fatphobia and transphobia that many women and people of marginalised genders encounter alongside it. But while it set out to highlight a problem and prove a point, it also showed me the power of sisterhood and solidarity when it comes to finding solutions.

'I thought I was the only one.' 'I thought I was going mad.' 'I thought maybe I was just weak.' I'm constantly horrified by just how frequently I hear phrases like this when it comes to women's health. Too often, women are left isolated, confused and disempowered by paternalistic 'doctor knows best' attitudes that discount the knowledge and expertise they have about their bodies. It's not just research, knowledge and understanding that's sorely lacking in so many areas of women's health; there's also an issue with empathy and trust. But, when medicine treats women as unreliable witnesses to their own suffering, there are growing communities of activists and advocates forming to fill the void.

From periods and gynae health, to chronic pain, mental health and disability, there have never been more pockets of the internet – or, indeed, the offline world – dedicated to awareness raising and peer support. These are places where women and other marginalised people can find information, advice and, above all, reassurance that they're not alone.

Many of those who submit blog posts to Hysterical Women have found it through this kind of 21st-century consciousness raising. Some have started petitions or campaigns or formed their own community support groups. Many more have made a difference to someone in their life simply by speaking out and telling their own story – only to experience the snowball effect of friends and relatives responding with, 'Oh my god, that happened to me too!'

In 2020 I also launched #ShitMyDoctorSays, an Instagram series of things that healthcare professionals have actually said out loud to their patients and, occasionally, to their colleagues. It's been a powerful way of highlighting some of the more explicit examples of medical misogyny – a shareable, micro version of Hysterical Women, featuring quotes like 'The pain is all in your head' and 'You're a woman, deal with it.'

I've shared dozens and dozens of these comments, but they still continue to shock me. Although they're always anonymised,

I'm continually struck by how similar and universal they are. Regardless of the context or the condition, so many of these remarks could have come straight out of a book of unhelpful and insensitive medical phrases. I'm sure 'How to fob off your patients' isn't actually a module in medical school, yet many healthcare professionals appear to have developed a strikingly similar technique.

*

While many of these stories are critical of the words and actions of individual doctors, the issues at play are, of course, structural and systemic. I have always been a huge advocate of the NHS and, like so many of us, am indebted to its care. But, like healthcare systems globally, it is not without its faults.

Some of these exist simply by virtue of it being an organisation made up of human beings – with all the skills, flaws, positive qualities and prejudices that every human being brings to their work. But, while every healthcare professional has some personal responsibility for their own practice, it's also vital that we explore these issues in the context of a health service under enormous pressure.

Even before the Covid-19 pandemic, the NHS had experienced a decade of austerity measures and under-resourcing. A 2017 report by the King's Fund, the charity that works to improve health and care in the UK, states that: 'The NHS is under growing financial pressure. Between 2010/11 and 2014/15, health spending increased by an average of 1.2 per cent a year in real terms… This is far below the annual growth rate of 3.7 per cent in previous years and is not sufficient to cover growing demand.'

This slowdown in funding growth, it concluded, was 'increasing the pressure on staff' and 'storing up problems for the future.' These problems have, of course, been all too apparent since the outbreak of Covid-19, with high levels of staff burnout reported, as well as significant disruption to healthcare services. According to a report by the doctors' professional body, the

British Medical Association (BMA), published in July 2020, much of this was 'avoidable'.

It states, 'Although a pandemic on the scale of Covid-19 was always likely to cause major disruption to health services, the drastic extent to which the NHS had to shut down routine care is a consequence of over a decade of underinvestment and (in the case of public health and social care) cuts to services.'

As a result, the report continues, NHS capacity lagged behind that of many EU countries, including in terms of bed numbers, critical care facilities, workforce numbers (with 10,000 NHS medical vacancies in England in 2019), and resources in primary and community care. 'The NHS was already in crisis before the pandemic hit, as the BMA consistently warned,' the report writers add. Even now, it is unclear exactly what post-Covid NHS recovery will look like and how long it is likely to take.

But what does this big picture stuff have to do with gender and other biases? Pressures on the NHS, both pre- and post-pandemic, undoubtedly affect all patients to some extent. However, women are the biggest users of health and social care services, both for themselves and as parents and carers, so they inevitably feel the biggest impact of under-resourcing.

For many, this begins as early as adolescence, with problematic periods, the burden of responsibility for contraception, and later cervical screening creating additional 'health admin', even for otherwise young and healthy women. Where a typical 25-year-old cis woman may visit her GP twice a year for a pill check, or every few years for a coil change or smear test, many typical 25-year-old cis men may only have attended a handful of times since childhood. The disruption to GP, sexual health and screening services has therefore had a much more widespread impact on women and those assigned female at birth than their otherwise young and healthy male peers – the majority of whom have, presumably, barely noticed any difference.

We also know the pandemic has exacerbated many of the social determinants of health, with issues like poverty, working conditions, job insecurity and housing all key drivers of health inequalities. This means the indirect health impacts of the pandemic, including on mental health and food poverty, have fallen hardest on marginalised groups. Again, research shows disruption to routine healthcare appointments, prescriptions and procedures during the pandemic disproportionately affected women, older people and minority ethnic groups.

Resourcing issues aside, our existing medical model has not served us well since long before Covid-19. When you add in the historic exclusion of women from medical trials, the underfunding of research into women's health issues, and the several thousand years' worth of conscious and unconscious bias, it's clear that the system was designed by and for white, cisgender men. It's not hard to see why women and other marginalised groups might fare worse in a system that's stacked against us – particularly when that system is so desperately struggling for the time and resources necessary to provide a high standard of care.

From medical research and education through to policy and management, gaps in knowledge, understanding, representation, trust and funding leave women and other marginalised groups at risk of poorer health outcomes and poorer care. Experiences like those shared on Hysterical Women and #ShitMyDoctorSays shine a light on the myriad ways these inequalities manifest in practice and the enormous impact they have on real people's lives. Of course, it shouldn't be up to women to fix centuries' worth of systemic medical misogyny and bias, but I do believe our influence is vital.

✳

People often ask me how I ended up writing about these issues. They often assume I have endometriosis or myalgic encephalomyelitis/chronic fatigue syndrome (ME/CFS) – two of the conditions I'm most vocal about – but I don't. In many respects, I've been lucky really. My health is generally good, although I have ongoing struggles with depression, anxiety and post-traumatic stress disorder (PTSD). I'm also very fortunate to have two extremely supportive female GPs at my local surgery – although they're used to me turning up to consultations having already pitched, researched and interviewed a specialist for an article on whatever issue I'm there to discuss with them.

That said, I've also experienced my share of feeling dismissed or fobbed off by healthcare professionals. A consultant neurologist told me, nine months after I fractured two vertebrae in a car accident, that losing weight would probably fix my persistent back pain. I was a UK size 10–12 at the time, in too much pain to exercise and it still took months before anyone actually referred me for the physiotherapy I needed.

When I came off the pill after 10 years, my menstrual cycles were so irregular for such a long time afterwards that I was investigated for polycystic ovary syndrome (PCOS). I don't have PCOS, but I later learned that this phenomenon is sometimes referred to as 'post-pill PCOS' and, in my case, it took almost two years for my cycles to settle back down into some kind of post-pill normality. Yet when I asked a dermatologist to prescribe a non-hormonal alternative for my acne, he repeatedly dismissed and ignored my concerns, telling me to just go back on the pill until I wanted to get pregnant and adding that my acne would probably improve during pregnancy anyway.

In the end I got my way. He prescribed topical treatments, which did exactly what I wanted them to do, providing a long-term fix that didn't keep me held hostage to hormones. But it shouldn't have been such a fight to be heard – or, indeed, to access treatments that are presumably first-line options for male patients.

Despite these and other examples, the honest answer is that I fell into this work almost by accident. After years of writing about all aspects of women's mental, physical and sexual health, I was increasingly pissed off about hearing the same stories of mistreatment and dismissal over and over again. I was frustrated by how little medical science seemed to know about conditions that predominantly affect women and baffled that no one was funding research into subjects that were fascinating to me. As a feminist it was this sense of injustice, rather than my own personal experience, that lit a fire under me.

However, a month or so into writing this book, I also found out I was pregnant – which has certainly added a more personal dimension. Much of chapter 8, 'Baby blues', was aptly written and edited through a haze of first trimester nausea, anxiety and exhaustion. By the time these words reach you that little embryo, gestated alongside this book, will be a fully-fledged miniature human being. And so this work has taken on an extra layer of significance – a hope for the future, that his generation will both benefit from and continue to build upon the gender health gap revolution that's recorded here.

Much has started to be written in recent years about the gender pain gap, medical gaslighting and broader inequalities in health. Research has shown time and time again that this is a problem and the wider medical community is slowly starting to wake up to it. This book is not about proving that the problem exists or persuading you that you should care. It does and you should. Instead, what I'm interested in exploring is the impact on real patients' lives, where we go from here, and how patient advocacy and activism is leading the way.

Many of the campaigners and communities featured in this book are women, trans men and non-binary individuals who have influenced so much of my work over the years. I hope their stories reassure, enrage and inspire you as much as they have done me. It's worth pointing out, though, that these stories represent some of the worst examples of medical practice. Many more of us will have had much more positive experiences of the hard-working, compassionate people who work within the NHS. The aim of this book isn't to frighten you, or put you off accessing care, but to highlight the systemic issues at play and hopefully empower you with the tools to join the fightback in whatever way works for you.

I want to show that healthcare activism and advocacy comes in many forms, not all of which need to be big, loud and visible. Often there is a quiet power simply in informing yourself, speaking out and sharing your story – whether that's with one other person or a million of them. I also want to highlight how intimately connected all of these issues are. I've tried to include a diverse and intersectional range of voices and experiences throughout, although I'm aware there will inevitably be gaps. I have never believed that the struggles of women and the (often intersecting) struggles of other marginalised groups are mutually exclusive or at odds with each other. We are all fighting a common enemy and have so much around which to unite, although our experiences, struggles, privileges and oppressions may be very different.

Ultimately, this book tells the story of the gender health gap from the perspective of all those many, many real women, and others, whose voices and stories too often remain hidden behind the scenes. These are the people who are living it, speaking out about it and leading the long overdue revolution in healthcare by creating a manifesto for change.

2

'Some girls just have bad periods': Menstrual and hormonal health

For most girls, starting your period (officially known as menarche) is a defining moment, although exactly what it means will vary from one person to the next. It's an event surrounded by cliches about 'becoming a woman' – invoking pride and a feeling of 'grown-up-ness' for some, while for others it's a source of shame, anxiety, confusion, embarrassment and pain.

Of course, not all girls and women do menstruate, and not everyone who menstruates is a girl or woman – and falling into either of these camps comes with its own complex set of feelings and challenges. One in every 5000 girls will be born with Mayer Rokitansky Küster Hauser syndrome (MRKH), a congenital abnormality resulting in a shortened vagina and an absent cervix and womb. Most of these girls will only discover they have MRKH during puberty, when they experience all the other typical changes but don't start having periods. Another one in 10,000 girls and young women will be affected by premature ovarian insufficiency (POI), or premature menopause, under the age of 20, where their periods either never start or disappear in the first few years after making an entrance.

For these young women, as well as for trans girls, the absence of periods can be a source of intense grief – a reckoning with their own body and fertility, and a defining feature that marks them out from their peers. Similarly, for trans boys and non-binary young people who were assigned female at birth, the arrival of menstruation can be a distressing source of gender dysphoria and discomfort, and a feeling of being betrayed by their own body.

Even for the majority of girls and young women who experience menarche as expected, the arrival of a monthly cycle is not without baggage. There's a whole mythology surrounding periods and their symptoms – from acne and mood swings related to pre-menstrual syndrome (PMS) to abdominal and breast pain. This, we're told, is the curse of Eve; a woman's lot is to suffer, and we might as well suck it up and get used to it now. For many of us these symptoms will be mild and manageable with over-the-counter pain relief, a hot water bottle and a family-size bar of chocolate, but for many more this will be the start of a decades-long battle with reproductive health and healthcare.

Given the uterine origins of 'hysteria', it's perhaps unsurprising that a huge number of the stories submitted to Hysterical Women relate in some way to the menstrual cycle, from reproductive health issues like endometriosis, fibroids and PCOS to cyclical hormonal issues like pre-menstrual dysphoric disorder (PMDD), the severe form of PMS.

I hear from women – and, to a lesser extent, trans men and non-binary people – whose often-debilitating symptoms have been repeatedly dismissed by their doctors as 'normal'; something that anyone with a womb simply has to put up with. This is where the 'periods = suffering' myth becomes so dangerous. All of the symptoms associated with monthly hormone fluctuations exist on a spectrum, ranging from normal and manageable through to abnormal and symptomatic of a deeper issue. But the idea that all period-related pain and suffering is simply 'to be expected' too often becomes a barrier to accessing appropriate and available care.

In her iconic 1978 essay, 'If Men Could Menstruate', feminist Gloria Steinem imagines a world in which only men have periods. Periods, she writes, 'would become an enviable, boast-worthy, masculine event.' She imagines cis men bragging about the flow and duration of their periods; society treating both menarche and menopause as events to be publicly marked and celebrated; and menstruation being used to justify men's superior position in war, politics and religion. She envisages free, federally funded pads and tampons and, she says, 'To prevent monthly work loss among the powerful, Congress would fund a National Institute of Dysmenorrhea [period pain].' Imagine that!

Almost 40 years later, there are still gaping holes in medical research's understanding of common period issues, never mind anything more complex. Research shows that more than 50% of young women experience period pain bad enough to need medication, yet the medications used to treat period pain (oral contraceptives and non-steroidal anti-inflammatories like ibuprofen) have a 20–25% failure rate.

A 2016 review, oft-cited by women's health activists and advocates, also found that researchers conduct five times as many studies into erectile dysfunction (ED) as PMS, despite the former affecting just 19% of men while the latter, in varying forms, affects 90% of women. An earlier review found that 40% of women with PMS do not respond to any of the currently available treatments. Meanwhile, men with ED can now readily buy Viagra over the counter in UK pharmacies.

I could easily have filled an entire book on the problems, and the patient advocacy, surrounding menstrual and hormonal health. It has been a huge hot topic in recent years, and an exciting and dynamic new wave of feminist health activism has emerged from the simple everyday activism of people shunning period taboos and speaking out about their monthly experiences. For the purpose of this chapter, though, I've focused on the conditions that crop up most frequently on Hysterical Women and in my broader work: endometriosis, fibroids, PMDD and PCOS. While not exhaustive by any means, the experiences and the activism of patients with these conditions cover a lot of common ground.

*

Endometriosis always feels like the most obvious starting point for any conversation about gender bias and inequalities in healthcare. In fact, it was writing an article on endometriosis that first inspired me to start digging further into these issues, long before I realised quite how deep they go. Endometriosis is the second most common gynaecological condition, after uterine fibroids, and affects an estimated one in 10 women and people assigned female at birth (AFAB). It's a chronic inflammatory condition, where tissue similar to the uterine lining (the endometrium) is found outside the womb, most commonly attaching itself to the other organs in the pelvis.

As such, it can cause symptoms that include agonisingly painful or heavy periods, pain during sex, infertility or fertility issues, and bladder or bowel problems, as well as chronic pelvic and abdominal pain, bloating (known as 'endo belly') and fatigue. These symptoms can be debilitating and, as I mentioned earlier, endometriosis costs the UK economy £8.2 billion a year in treatment, loss of work and healthcare costs.

Despite this, and the fact that it affects roughly as many women as diabetes, medical science still does not know what causes the condition and there is no cure. Endometriosis can currently only be diagnosed via laparoscopic surgery and the gold standard treatment is excision surgery to remove the tissue. Even this is no panacea; relief is often short-lived and there's such a shortage of specialists that access to surgery is typically something of a postcode lottery. Instead, many patients spend years on the contraceptive pill, or other hormonal contraceptives, without even a diagnosis.

Unsurprisingly, a 2020 study into gender disparities in health research funding highlighted that endometriosis and other female-dominant conditions are among the worst funded by the US National Institutes of Health, while health issues that predominantly affect men are, of course, over-funded. This lack of medical knowledge, combined with its association with the womb and 'women's troubles', makes endometriosis one of the archetypal 'hysterical' conditions.

Its sufferers are dismissed, ignored, disbelieved and fobbed off to such an extent that it takes an average of eight years to be diagnosed with endometriosis in the UK. As recently as 2017 the National Institute for Health and Care Excellence (NICE), the public body that provides advice on improving health and social care in England, published its first guidance on endometriosis, including advice for doctors to 'listen to women'. Yet I've heard from women who waited more than two decades for a diagnosis; who were repeatedly told by doctors that their symptoms were 'just a bad period' or 'all in your head', or else were misdiagnosed with irritable bowel syndrome (IBS), depression or anxiety and sent on their merry way.

Dee Montague experienced all of these and more during her 23-year journey to a diagnosis. Writing for Hysterical Women, she draws a comparison between her experiences of asthma and endometriosis. 'Fun fact: I was born with asthma and no healthcare professional has ever, ever suggested my asthma symptoms were normal, psychosomatic or something I just had to put up with. Nor have I ever been denied medication or treatment pathways,' she says.

'My experience as an asthma patient is brilliant. My treatment is almost entirely patient-led, I have regular reviews, and healthcare professionals almost always understand what asthma is and how it can affect patients. My symptoms and how I deal with them are not viewed as a character flaw. How I wish I could say the same for my menstrual health.'

Dee goes on to describe the countless appointments, contraceptives, blood tests, sexually transmitted infection tests, misdiagnoses and even surgeries she went through before paying privately to see an endometriosis specialist. It was only then, more than 20 years after her agonising periods first began, that she was finally diagnosed with extensive stage 4 endometriosis, as well as adenomyosis, the even less well-known sister condition of endometriosis, which affects the muscle fibres inside the womb.

Dee is far from the only woman I've heard from who resorted to going private in order to get answers and treatment, but it's not something that everyone can afford to do, or that anyone should have to. Many, like Isabel Dunmore, simply give up, feeling they've exhausted all their options. 'After three and a half years of actively trying to seek help, explaining my symptoms and history to multiple doctors, and going for all kinds of tests and scans, I had given up,' she writes.

'I gave up on finding out why I was bent over in pain all the time, why I had long, heavy and erratic periods, why at times I'd lost control of my bowels, felt like I could pass out from fatigue and heavy blood loss, or why my body let me down for days, after nights spent curled up with pain.'

Instead, she convinced herself that maybe it really was all in her head after all. 'Maybe this is what every woman goes through and my pain tolerance is just really low. It's normal, right?' she says. 'So, I carried on, managing as best I could, accepting that some days I would be bedridden, unable to see my friends or do my usual activities. Some days I would drag myself out of bed to commute to work and sit in agony at my desk all day, forcing a smile.'

In the end, Isabel's endometriosis diagnosis happened 'almost by accident' five years later, during surgery to remove an ovarian cyst the size of a tennis ball. Even this had initially been misdiagnosed as appendicitis, despite her history of reproductive health concerns.

✽

'So often we see menstrual health issues being normalised – people are told they're making it up or they're being a wuss or they just have to put up with it,' says Emma Cox, CEO of Endometriosis UK. 'Why do we assume everyone's periods are going to be the same? We're all different shapes and sizes, our eyes aren't identical, our breasts aren't identical, why would our wombs and gynaecological health be?'

For her, part of the problem is treating menstrual pain by simply sticking young women straight on the pill. 'We seem to medicate with hormones without investigations to find the underlying cause. The pill can be a treatment for endometriosis symptoms, although it doesn't get rid of the disease, but with what other condition would we medicate someone for 10 years without looking for the cause, or even letting them know there might be an underlying cause?' she says. 'It just shows menstrual issues are not a priority.'

What patients really need, Emma adds, is the development of a non-surgical diagnostic test, better guidelines on pain management and improved access to specialist endometriosis centres – not to mention major investment into researching causes, treatment options and, ultimately, cures. All of this must go hand in hand with improved training and education for doctors, and a massive cultural shift in the way menstrual health is regarded.

Over the years, women have repeatedly told me about doctors dismissing their pain as 'all psychological'. Many are told that 'some girls just have bad periods' – a message they internalise and believe for years afterwards, putting them off continuing to seek help until their symptoms become unbearable. One even told me about being refused painkillers and accused of 'drug-seeking' when attending A&E in agony, only to witness a man in the next bay being prescribed morphine for his gallstone pain. Some have had doctors simply laugh in their faces or tell them to 'suck it up' and stop exaggerating their pain.

One of the most shocking stories ever submitted to #ShitMyDoctorSays was from a female medic with endometriosis. 'I worked in theatres and heard this directly from a surgeon's mouth. He hated doing the laparoscopy list querying endometriosis, because, he said, "They're all f*cking mental,"' she writes. 'Disheartening to witness, and even more so for the unconscious patient who'd misplaced their trust in a biased medical professional, who had already written them off before the anaesthetic.'

For many decades endometriosis also suffered from the misconception that it was a career women's disease – specifically one affecting white, high-earning, middle class women who chose to delay having children. It's possible this was largely driven by the fact these were the only patients with sufficient time, status and resources to successfully fight for a diagnosis. But it's also hard to miss the ancient echoes of hysteria in the implication that, by neglecting their childbearing duties, women had brought their illness upon themselves.

Although the idea has largely been debunked, I still routinely hear from people who have been advised by their doctor to 'just get pregnant' as if this were a) an easy option and b) a cure (it isn't). It's also a misconception that continues to harm women of colour with endometriosis, like Fiona Timba who runs the Instagram account @EndoSoBlack. 'Historically, endometriosis was perceived as a "white women's disease". Doctors believed it was less common in Black women, when the reality was actually that Black women's pain is often ignored by medical professionals,' she writes.

Instead, she adds, doctors often misdiagnosed endometriosis as fibroids – benign uterine growths that cause heavy, painful periods and abdominal pain or bloating, which are two to three times more common in Black women than white women. Another common misdiagnosis, Fiona says, was pelvic inflammatory disease (PID) – a painful condition typically caused by a sexually transmitted bacterial infection – as doctors believed Black women were more 'sexually promiscuous' than white women.

It took 13 years for Fiona to be diagnosed with endometriosis. 'When I look back on my experiences with doctors, I can't help but feel angry and let down now I understand the reasons for their questions, challenges and pushback on my attempts to get help,' she says. 'Black women shouldn't have to fight to have our pain heard or believed.'

For patients who experience this kind of racial bias, though, it's often easier not to mention it than risk care being withdrawn, says fellow endometriosis sufferer Saschan Fearon-Josephs. 'The issues around structural racism in the NHS massively trickle down to the way patients are treated. But if you bring it up, sometimes the person you're raising it with will end up gaslighting you into believing their racism is all in your head,' she says. 'When you're at the point of asking for healthcare, you're already vulnerable. I've been in situations where I felt like I didn't have any choice but to accept it.'

*

Another worrying thread that runs through endometriosis care – and, indeed, care for other reproductive health issues – is an apparent eagerness among some gynaecological surgeons to whip women's uteruses out at the drop of a hat. A hysterectomy is not a cure for endometriosis, although it can be, as a last resort, for conditions like adenomyosis, PMDD and fibroids. Yet all too often I hear from women, many of them young and still hoping to start a family one day, who've been advised to have this major, life-changing surgery as a first-line treatment.

Aimee (not her real name), at the age of 23, was offered a hysterectomy as an alternative to waiting 10 months for excision surgery on the NHS. 'I felt I was offered it before they'd even properly examined my endometriosis – really not an appropriate way to shrug off women with chronic illnesses,' she tells me. 'I said I wanted to at least try excision surgery before being fobbed off with a hysterectomy, but they just sort of shrugged and said it was the end of my options.'

Instead, Aimee sought the advice of a private specialist, who explained that a hysterectomy wouldn't have helped because endometriosis grows outside the womb. In her case it was also very extensive – growing on her bowel, bladder, and in her ligaments and hips – and she's since had multiple surgeries to remove it. 'Just imagine if I hadn't had the funds to go privately, and was so desperate to get rid of the daily pain and trauma that I'd agreed to a hysterectomy,' she says, looking back.

For Kim Salmons it was a private gynaecologist who recommended a total hysterectomy as first-line treatment for a large fibroid. Kim's surgeon proposed removing everything from her cervix to her ovaries – a procedure that would have plunged her into a surgical menopause more than a decade before she'd go through it naturally.

'I just took him at his word. I don't know why I didn't look into it further – I'm a researcher – but I absolutely trusted him,' she says. 'It was only when a couple of friends said, "Are you sure?" that I started reading up on it.' Having done her research, Kim opted instead for a uterine artery embolisation procedure to shrink the fibroid. When her symptoms returned after five years of relief, she eventually opted for a much less radical partial hysterectomy, leaving her cervix and ovaries intact. 'The surgeon I saw that time was much more gentle. She explained everything and she totally understood why I didn't want everything removing unnecessarily.'

Similarly, Roxanne Escobales was advised to have a hysterectomy to treat the large fibroid that she describes as her 'vampire baby'. 'It makes me look and feel pregnant because it's so big. It drains all of my energy, and I'm constantly in a state of low-level pain and discomfort,' she says.

In her case, the justification for a hysterectomy was that she was too old – no longer of 'child-bearing' age – for it to be worth trying other options, such as a myomectomy or embolisation, to remove or shrink the fibroids. 'I guess a myomectomy is a more challenging surgery for them, for someone who's not of childbearing age, but I was quite shocked by the idea of a hysterectomy. It felt like an extreme suggestion and I didn't act on it for about a year,' she says. 'In the end I just got fed up with living like this though.'

At the other end of the spectrum there are those who desperately do want a hysterectomy, but have to beg and plead to be allowed the surgery. Alex (not their real name), who is non-binary, tells me they had always felt a lot of discomfort and dysphoria about their uterus, made worse by the severe endometriosis and adenomyosis they'd suffered with since their teens.

'For a long time gynaecologists were very dismissive, saying the pain was all in my head, because of my history of mental health issues. When I finally got my laparoscopy and excision surgery, the surgeon was very apologetic – I was totally riddled with endometriosis,' they say. Over the following few years, Alex tried every treatment going, including further surgeries, but nothing worked. By this point they were bed-bound, sleeping 16 hours a day and unable to work. At their wit's end, they started pushing for a hysterectomy – which would at least rid them of adenomyosis – but met endless roadblocks.

'I'd first mentioned a hysterectomy in my teens and I'd always said I didn't want children, so this wasn't a new thing that I'd plucked out of thin air,' they say. 'I was told I was too young; I'd need to be cleared by psychiatry; I needed to see another pain specialist; and I'd have to freeze eggs even though I knew I'd never use them. It took a hell of a long time – years of arguing and fighting – for my surgeon to finally agree to do the hysterectomy.'

In many ways all these experiences are two sides of the same bodily autonomy coin: our wombs, our bodies even, are not our own. Just as in reproductive and perinatal health, there's an underlying idea that doctors are better placed than us to make informed decisions about our bodies and that those decisions can be dictated to us by our age, our fertility status, our anatomy or our gender.

It's also worth pointing out that for trans men and non-binary people affected by any of these menstrual health issues, accessing healthcare comes with the additional baggage of navigating a system steeped in the language of 'women's health' and 'womanhood', from which they may feel excluded or unwelcome.

*

June-Ann Joseph lives with PCOS, a condition that affects around one in 10 women and AFAB people. PCOS is a complex endocrine disorder (meaning it's related to the glands that release hormones into the blood), typically characterised by irregular periods, high levels of androgens causing excess facial or body hair (hirsutism) and enlarged (polycystic) ovaries containing fluid-filled follicles. Other symptoms include thinning hair, oily or acne-prone skin and weight gain due to insulin resistance – but more than 50% of people with PCOS won't have any symptoms.

For June-Ann, getting a diagnosis was the easy part, but, she says, any kind of aftercare has been severely lacking. 'I was given a pamphlet, but the GP said she didn't recommend going on birth control as I was still having regular periods. In my mind, for more than a decade afterwards, this was just a gynaecological problem and, as long as my periods weren't irregular, it wasn't causing any problems.'

Over the following years, June-Ann experienced a range of physical and mental health symptoms, including changes to her hair, weight gain, bouts of depression and anxiety, and very heavy, prolonged periods – but neither she nor her doctors ever connected the dots. Instead, she was prescribed antidepressants or, most frequently, told that losing weight would solve her problems.

It wasn't until 2020, at the age of 31, that June-Ann discovered the PCOS 'Cysterhood' on Instagram and started to really understand the extent of the ways in which her condition affects her – not through highly trained medical professionals, but through other patients sharing information and resources online. 'It made me realise that my anxiety and all these other issues were so closely linked with my PCOS. I honestly believe the gaps in my care were just because GPs don't know enough about my condition,' she says.

'Things like the weight stigma I experienced are very common in the community and it just makes you feel like shit.' Although research does show that weight loss can improve PCOS symptoms, the dismissive attitudes she and others experience feel especially unfair given the Catch-22 that PCOS itself contributes to weight gain and makes weight loss more difficult.

'No doctor ever actually worked with me on a care plan to help me lose weight; they just told me that was the problem and sent me away. Because they weren't connecting the dots between PCOS and my weight, they seemed to look at me and assume I was just lazy or not trying hard enough,' she says.

Health journalist Lydia Smith has also suffered from anxiety for many years. When she started experiencing other symptoms, like facial hair, weight gain and night sweats – which impacted on her body image – her GP suggested PCOS and sent her for investigations. But Lydia's subsequent healthcare experiences have left her feeling frustrated.

'My blood test results showed low oestrogen and my ultrasound showed an enlarged ovary, both of which suggest PCOS, so I was referred to a gynaecologist,' she says. 'His response felt very dismissive. He basically said there wasn't a lot they could do for my symptoms, but that if I wanted to have children then I should get on with it – otherwise, just take the pill.'

When Lydia explained that, like many women, she'd previously experienced distressing mental health side-effects on the pill, her gynaecologist seemed nonplussed. Equally, when she explained that she did want children one day, but wasn't ready yet, his advice was: 'Don't push it.'

'There was no concern about whether it was affecting my mental health – despite the fact research shows women with PCOS are more likely to be diagnosed with depression, anxiety or bipolar,' Lydia says. 'Even just some acknowledgement and validation that, "Yes, it can affect your mental health, you're not going mad," would have helped.'

Likewise, she says, despite the increased risk of type 2 diabetes and cardiovascular disease that comes with having PCOS, she has never been offered any guidance about managing her symptoms through diet and lifestyle changes. 'I've had to manage as best I can by doing my own research, which feels like that standard thing where women have to take their health into their own hands. There's a lot of rubbish information out there too, which just makes it harder to know what you can trust,' Lydia says.

What's most frustrating, she adds, is that 'Every doctor I've spoken to has said, "Oh it's so common." If it's so common, why the hell don't we know anything about it? If it affected this many men, we would have endless research. We would have treatment options. We would at the very least have more information widely available about managing it. But, because it's a reproductive issue, it's just brushed under the carpet.'

The only exception to this seems to be if you're struggling to conceive, Lydia says – a comment I've also heard repeated by women with endometriosis. 'It just makes you feel like a handmaid; that somebody is only listening to you when it's about having kids. It was only when I mentioned that I was thinking about starting a family that I felt like they were taking me seriously. Otherwise, you're on your own. They don't seem to be interested in your mental health, the facial hair, the weight gain. You're just left to get on with it.'

*

As with the varying attitudes towards hysterectomy, treatment discussions around PCOS seem to return again and again to gendered assumptions about the patient's sexuality, fertility or family plans. Neelam Heera, who was diagnosed with PCOS while at university, describes how attitudes about hormonal contraception commonly act as a barrier to treatment in British Asian communities. When her own South Asian GP prescribed the contraceptive pill to treat her symptoms, he added, 'Just because you're on the pill, doesn't mean you can go sleeping around!'

'It was a comment I just accepted, because most Asian males have this attitude,' she says. In fact, some men in Neelam's family took even less kindly to her treatment. 'My uncles were fuming when they found out I was on the contraceptive pill. They didn't ask why. They were just pissed off and to this day don't speak to me. They didn't see it as me taking medication, they saw it as me being sexually promiscuous,' she explains. This, Neelam adds, poses a serious problem for many British Asians living with reproductive health issues, particularly given the current lack of alternative options.

Fellow South Asian Riz had the opposite problem. As a non-binary person in a relationship with a cis woman, their doctor told them there was no point prescribing the pill as a treatment for their PCOS and suspected endometriosis, because they didn't need it for contraception. 'I had to really push to go on the combined pill just to stop me being in pain every time I got my period,' they say. While their doctor did eventually, reluctantly, prescribe the pill, it again highlights the conflation by many in the medical profession of menstrual health with sexuality and reproduction.

The lack of alternatives also poses the risk of desperate patients – particularly those from communities with plenty of reason to distrust colonial Western medicine – turning to unregulated, and potentially dangerous, wellness 'remedies'. Traditional practices like yoni (vaginal) steaming have a long cultural history in parts of Africa, Asia and Central America, although they've more recently been made famous (not to mention controversial and expensive) by wellness brands like Gwyneth Paltrow's Goop. But while there's only anecdotal evidence to suggest these practices offer any tangible health benefits, the risks include burns, allergic reactions and vaginal infections, as well as induced miscarriage. One woman, who I interviewed in 2019, told me she'd started looking into the traditional techniques used by her Caribbean ancestors after realising the pill isn't a cure or long-term solution for PCOS, simply a way of masking the symptoms.

These frustrations are understandable and, of course, a big part of the problem is a lack of research funding to find alternatives. 'There are lots of good ideas floating around, but funding is an issue,' says Professor Stephen Franks, a professor of reproductive endocrinology at Imperial College London. Equally, where treatments do exist – like topical creams to reduce hair growth – GPs are often reluctant to prescribe them because of the cost.

'Funding for ovulatory disorders, and women's health generally, is pretty poor. We haven't seen any radical changes in management and we certainly don't have a treatment that will reverse all the effects of polycystic ovary syndrome,' he says. 'I have a colleague in the US who's very prominent in the world of PCOS, but when she applies for grants it's on the theme of metabolic disorders, because PCOS is not thought to be a priority.'

That said, Stephen does believe there have been improvements in GP awareness of the condition and an increase in referrals to specialists. 'It does seem to be improving gradually, and patient power is very important for making those in primary care sit up and pay attention,' he says. 'Organisations like PCOS charity Verity can help you to become well informed and even find the name of a specialist locally who you can ask to be referred to. Often, I think GPs will be quite relieved if you can provide this kind of information.'

★

Just as the physical symptoms of menstrual health issues have been normalised for centuries, so too have the psychological effects. PMS affects virtually all people who menstruate to some extent or another and covers a huge range of symptoms, including mood swings, depression, irritability, cravings, disrupted sleep, breast tenderness and headaches. Just like pain and menstrual flow, PMS symptoms exist on a spectrum, ranging from normal and manageable to abnormal and debilitating.

Severe PMS, known as PMDD, is estimated to affect 5–8% of women and people who menstruate, or roughly 800,000 people in the UK. Like endometriosis, many sufferers go years without ever even hearing of PMDD, let alone being diagnosed with it. This lack of awareness is compounded by the shadow of hysteria; the received wisdom that our wombs can literally drive us to madness. But PMS that leaves you contemplating suicide – as, at its most extreme, PMDD can – is never normal and should never be dismissed as such.

In 2017 I interviewed Sarah, who suffered from such severe PMDD that, at the age of just 23, she faced a stark, life-changing choice between her mental health and sacrificing her fertility for a hysterectomy and oopherectomy (removal of the ovaries).

Since the age of 14 she'd experienced disturbing images and voices during the fortnight before each period, as well as hypermania, mania, depression and suicidal ideation. At their worst, these monthly episodes led her to terrifying situations where Sarah went missing for days at a time, was repeatedly hospitalised and even sectioned under the Mental Health Act. 'It's like sleep-walking into a car crash, but then my period will start, the symptoms will go away and I'll be really well in between times,' she told me.

Sarah's experience is a particularly extreme example, but it does powerfully illustrate how the experiences of those affected by severe pre-menstrual disorders go way beyond just 'normal PMS'. Despite this, patients face an uphill battle for awareness, understanding and treatment.

Business psychologist Clare Knox has lived with PMDD since coming off the pill in her mid to late 20s. She now runs Luna Hub, a safe space for sufferers of PMDD, and in 2021 we teamed up for a collaborative #ShitMyDoctorSays post. Some of the responses she collected from the Luna Hub community were horrifying, ranging from suicidal women being sent away without support, to comments like, 'Don't go killing anyone' and 'PMS isn't real, let alone PMDD.'

'Unfortunately, there's a lot of dismissal and medical gaslighting – people being told it's all in their head, or it's just PMS, or not being given the support for the lifelong journey that is PMDD,' Clare says. 'A lot of GPs and even specialists haven't heard of PMDD; they're not well-versed in hormonal health and so they don't necessarily have the knowledge to treat it appropriately,' she explains.

Nathalie Saunders self-diagnosed her PMDD thanks to the much-maligned power of Dr Google. She describes feeling dismissed and fobbed off by doctors for years, as well as being judged for her queer, polyamorous identity and her weight. Despite the contraceptive pill making her mental health worse, doctors tried her on pill after pill after pill, apparently unconcerned that it was causing Nathalie to spend four or more hours a day crying.

'I still to this day believe that, because of its cyclical nature, doctors have downplayed or dismissed my mental distress, believing I will ultimately come out of it. How bad did it have to get before they listened? And would it always be dismissed because it was associated with my period?' she says.

Like many of the women with PMDD who I've heard from, this treatment itself impacted on Nathalie's mental health, as well as her faith in the medical system. 'I'm constantly scared I will be seen as hysterical,' she says. 'I've noticed just how much my words are twisted in doctors' notes and reports, and how my physical appearance can affect an entire appointment outcome.'

*

The good news is that recent years have seen a huge explosion of period activism. Menstrual health issues, particularly endometriosis and PMDD, have benefitted from significant awareness-raising campaigns, largely thanks to the tireless campaigning, speaking out and hard work of charities, activists and patient advocates like those we've met in this chapter.

Campaigns have successfully ended the tampon tax and seen free period products introduced in schools. Start-ups, largely run by women, have begun filling gaps in the menstrual market – from sustainable, organic and reusable period products to innovative new ways of tackling pain. And a whole host of Instagram accounts, along with books like Emma Barnett's *Period: It's About Bloody Time* and Maisie Hill's *Period Power*, are challenging long-established narratives about our monthly cycles.

Having struggled with period pain and PMS herself, Maisie's message is one of empowering women and other menstruators to really get to know their own bodies and work with them. 'Part of the problem is our bodies are just seen as a bit of a nuisance – a reproductive system that's liable to go wrong,' she tells me. 'The education around this is woefully lacking and totally focused on avoiding unwanted pregnancy. That requires a paradigm shift, to go from managing the body to really embracing and understanding it.'

One campaign that has gone some way towards creating this shift was the petition for menstrual health education started by Endometriosis UK trustee Alice Smith. After gaining more than 100,000 signatures, the petition was influential in getting periods added to the curriculum in English schools, which Endometriosis UK and Alice hope will help 'educate a generation' about the difference between normal and abnormal period symptoms.

'I'd been working with Endometriosis UK since I was about 18 on educating and starting conversations. I'd done talks in schools myself, but when the PSHE [personal, social, health and economic education] curriculum came up for renewal, that felt like our time to start the petition,' Alice explains. 'I can't go into every school myself, but this is something that is standardised and consistent across the whole country. Through this hopefully we should be able to start conversations and dismantle taboos and misinformation. This isn't just a women's problem, or a problem for people who menstruate; it's a social justice problem.'

Endometriosis UK and other regional charities are now working towards the expansion of this to schools in Wales, Scotland and Northern Ireland. One of those charities, which has been campaigning for menstrual health education in Wales since 2018, is Fair Treatment for the Women of Wales (FTWW), where Dee Montague now works part-time.

After starting life as a Facebook group, FTWW has grown into a national charity, advising the Welsh Government on issues across the whole of women's health, including menstrual health, multiple miscarriages and the menopause, as well as chronic and autoimmune conditions. 'It's a kind of sisterhood really, all about empowering each other and then presenting evidence about our collective experiences. From the perspective of making a change, it's that evidence that's so compelling,' Dee and FTWW founder Debbie Shaffer tell me.

Saschan Fearon-Josephs is another activist who has been instrumental in opening up the menstrual health conversation. Saschan founded the Womb Room in 2011, initially as a personal blog, after being repeatedly dismissed with an enormous, potentially fatal ovarian cyst. The Womb Room has since evolved into a coaching and workplace consultancy business, as well as using social media and events to reach the wider public. 'We started delivering workshops in schools around reproductive wellbeing and menstrual health. Now we also coach individual women and work with companies, which helps to fund our work with young people,' she says.

'My idea was, I can't change the NHS because it's too big an institution, but what I can do is help people to understand their bodies more, understand their options for moving through the healthcare system and support them with the skills to advocate for themselves.'

Similarly, alongside Luna Hub, Clare Knox runs See Her Thrive, a business psychology consultancy specialising in menstrual and hormonal health. One of the biggest challenges, she says, is ensuring those living with PMDD receive appropriate care and support, without feeding into existing and deeply ingrained sexist stereotypes. From a feminist perspective, how do we acknowledge the very real impact of PMDD on sufferers' mental health without fuelling the idea that women's menstrual cycles make us irrational, overly emotional and less competent, trustworthy or reliable?

'It's very tricky, and there's a fine balance between support and what we don't want to do, which is victimise women and make them appear weak, powerless or incapable,' Clare says.

'This can be one of the unintended consequences of workplace policies like menstrual leave and could actually exacerbate gender inequality. For me it really comes down to treating all employees as individuals and taking a more flexible, human-centred approach to management.'

Meanwhile, Neelam Heera runs Cysters, a Birmingham-based, trans-inclusive charity supporting people from marginalised communities who are affected by reproductive health issues. A big part of her work involves working with cultural and religious community leaders, as well as local NHS services, to bridge some of the gaps in understanding.

'Women from these communities carry the cultural attitudes, stigma and shame we've been raised with. From that perspective, accessing healthcare services as a person of colour is harder,' Neelam says. 'There's a lot in the NHS about diversity training, but we also need healthcare professionals to have cultural sensitivity training, because some of the things that patients report to us often carry undertones of racism and bias.'

Equally important is Cysters' role in giving people from marginalised backgrounds a voice and a seat at the table in conversations around reproductive health. Having not seen anyone like herself involved in menstrual health spaces, Neelam has worked hard to ensure that British Asian voices are included and represented, both in media and political lobbying on these issues.

The same is true for June-Ann Joseph. 'As a young Black girl, I didn't know much. Coming into the [online PCOS] community has influenced my advocacy so much, but I also didn't see anyone else who looked like me or who understood my cultural background,' she says. As a result, she was inspired to start her podcast, Black, Broke and Anxious, exploring her own and other Black women's experiences with PCOS and mental health issues.

'Even just saying the word "period" is a huge taboo in African and Caribbean communities, so I wanted to change that and help other Black women to understand when they might need to ask for help,' she explains. In the 12 months since she started the podcast, June-Ann's seen a 'ripple effect' of friends and family opening up more about their reproductive health and asking her for advice.

✳

Beyond racial and cultural issues, it's clear there's also still a lot of work to be done to make gynaecology and menstrual healthcare, as well as the patient communities that surround them, much more inclusive of patients who are not women. While many groups are, like Cysters, explicitly trans-inclusive, this kind of policy is not always a given and the US-based EndoQueer community was set up to provide a dedicated safe space for queer, trans and non-binary patients and their experiences.

The importance of these kinds of communities is a remarkably common theme across so many different health issues, but particularly in menstrual and reproductive health. Instagram, TikTok and Twitter, and private Facebook groups, provide a mine of information for patients looking for answers, support and reassurance – or even self-diagnosing mystery symptoms. It's something I find simultaneously depressing and inspiring.

On the one hand, it's an incredible testament to the resilience and compassion of women and marginalised people that such networks exist. Alongside fighting their own battles, these individuals have come together to support others, sharing the expertise they've gleaned during the course of their own journeys, and offering practical tips and advice to those still in the dark about their symptoms and care. Phenomenal amounts of research go on behind the scenes, as patients educate not only themselves and their doctors about their condition, but also each other.

It's worth pointing out, though, that any community of laypeople is vulnerable to biases, inaccuracies and misinformation, and a certain degree of health literacy is necessary to safely navigate the frankly overwhelming volume of information that exists online. Instagram, in particular, is a huge market for less reputable corners of the multi-billion-dollar wellness industry. It's no coincidence that this industry primarily targets women, and one of my biggest concerns about the gender health gap is the risk that it will drive business to exploitative companies and practitioners peddling unregulated 'miracle cures' to vulnerable people who are desperate enough to try anything.

That said, at their best these communities are incredibly valuable for those without the resources – the time, research skills or access to academic journals – to seek out all this information for themselves. They're also a vital source of sisterhood and support for anyone feeling isolated by their condition or by their treatment at the hands of healthcare professionals.

I hope this book will offer similarly supportive and informative toolkits, because I know that, in our current, broken system, this is what patients are crying out for. The caveat, of course, is that none of this should be necessary. I don't believe the onus should ever be on women or marginalised groups to diagnose themselves or to fix the deeply ingrained systemic issues that we're talking about here.

During the launch of a report from the All-Party Parliamentary Group on Endometriosis in October 2020, then health minister with responsibility for women's health, Nadine Dorries, said that women have an obligation 'not to be fobbed off' by doctors – comments she repeated on BBC Radio 4's *Woman's Hour* the following year. While I've got absolutely nothing against empowering women to advocate for themselves, her words – coming from a minister with power to effect meaningful, structural change – simply smacked of victim-blaming.

Tellingly, her initial comments were made in response to – or rather, as a way of dodging – the question, 'When will the government commit to [the All-Party Parliamentary Group report's recommendation on] reducing diagnosis times [for endometriosis]?' The government is still, at the time of writing, yet to make a specific, targeted commitment, apparently intent on blaming patients instead and pushing an agenda of personal responsibility.

Women regularly ask me for advice on how to be better advocates for themselves and I'm always happy to share the tips I've picked up over the years. I've also included them in the toolkit sections at the end of each chapter. But not everyone has the privilege of being able to advocate for themselves at all and, for those who do, there's still no guarantee that speaking up and challenging your doctor's opinion will get you anywhere, because the balance of power is simply not in our favour.

Even the doctors who are well-informed and eager to help remain limited in what they can do. Dr Hannah Short is a GP specialising in premenstrual disorders and the menopause – a practice that's been shaped by her own patient experiences with PMDD, endometriosis, and surgical menopause following a hysterectomy and removal of both ovaries. While she says it's wonderful to see increased awareness of these conditions, the demoralising reality for her as a doctor is that the system simply does not allow her to provide the level of care she'd like.

'There's post after post on social media about how doctors need to be better trained in menopause, PMDD etc. and, yes, there's an issue here. However, there are now so many of us who have undertaken training in our own time, at our own expense, who desperately want to help, but we are constantly prevented from doing so as a result of commissioning decisions,' she says.

'I think sometimes there are unrealistic expectations about what you're actually able to do as a GP. Sometimes it's because the GP doesn't have the requisite knowledge, because we're trained as generalists and can't be specialists in everything, but often it's just because of limitations on your practice, like only having a 10-minute appointment or not being able to prescribe specific medications locally,' Hannah explains.

'Besides all those logistical issues, which are completely out of our control, there aren't always specialist services available for us to refer on to. These services just aren't prioritised,' she adds. 'GP education and access to services will not and cannot improve until female hormonal health is taken seriously by the system as whole.'

Data published in 2022 showed that waiting lists for gynaecology increased by 60% during the pandemic – more than any other medical specialty – with more than half a million patients waiting to be seen. Then President of the Royal College of Obstetricians and Gynaecologists (RCOG), Dr Edward Morris, told the *Guardian* this was down to doctors routinely dismissing women's health problems as 'benign' – leading to them being 'normalised' and deprioritised within the NHS.

So, while I would absolutely love to empower every single person reading this book to feel more confident and better equipped to self-advocate in medical appointments, I also need you to know that fixing the centuries-old gender health gap is not your responsibility. Regardless of what government ministers may think, any bad care you receive is never your fault. It's not because you didn't try hard enough, didn't get enough second opinions or didn't make enough complaints; it's because the system has failed you. Too many patients are forced, by necessity, to become experts in their own conditions – and advocates for their own care – because their doctors lack the relevant knowledge or resources to diagnose or treat them appropriately.

YOUR MENSTRUAL HEALTH TOOLKIT

When it comes to period symptoms, one key tip is to consistently track your cycle. Make a note of the dates, volume and duration of your flow, and any symptoms you experience throughout the month, including pre-menstrual and mid-cycle symptoms. You can do so using any number of cycle-tracking apps or a simple pen and paper diary. This not only provides detailed information for your GP, but can also help you get to know your body better, to notice any patterns and understand what is 'normal' or typical for you.

'It can be really helpful if you've done some prior research before seeing your GP, so you can enter the appointment from a position of power,' Saschan Fearon-Josephs says. 'Most GPs don't have a lot of training around reproductive and menstrual health conditions, so they don't necessarily always put the symptoms together. If you've tracked your symptoms and done a bit of research, it's much easier to go in and request something specific, like investigations for a particular condition.'

Equally, she adds, 'If you feel like you're not being taken seriously, go and seek a second opinion. A lot of people don't realise they can do that. You really do need a lot of resilience, though, because it's exhausting. If you want answers, you have to keep fighting.'

Saschan also recommends researching local specialists in your condition, not just general gynaecologists, and pushing for a specific referral if you find someone who seems to know their stuff. 'Use Facebook groups and online communities, and learn from the experiences of other people with your condition,' she adds.

For women's health practitioner Maisie Hill, there is also a place for making lifestyle changes or trying alternative and complementary therapies, but these should be just that: complementary to medical advice and treatment. 'I'm a fan of whatever works, and I think it's important to be dynamic and responsive to whatever someone's needs are,' she says. 'We need to be treating menstrual health issues more holistically, so it shouldn't just be seen as one or the other.'

Resources
- Black, Broke & Anxious – instagram.com/BlackBrokeA ndAnxiousPodcast
- British Fibroid Trust – britishfibroidtrust.org.uk
- Cysters – cysters.org
- Endometriosis UK – endometriosis-uk.org
- EndoQueer – endoqueer.com
- Endo Silence Scotland – instagram.com/EndoSilenceScot
- Endo So Black – instagram.com/EndoSoBlack
- Fair Treatment for the Women of Wales (FTWW) – ftww.org.uk

- International Association for Premenstrual Disorders (IAPMD) – iapmd.org
- Luna Hub – lunahub.net
- Maisie Hill – maisiehill.com
- MRKH Connect – mrkhconnect.co.uk
- National Association for Premenstrual Syndromes (NAPS) – pms.org.uk
- Period Positive – periodpositive.com
- Red Moon Gang – redmoongang.com
- The Womb Room – instagram.com/thewombroom
- Verity PCOS – verity-pcos.org.uk
- Vicious Cycle PMDD – viciouscyclepmdd.com

3

'Attention-seeking hypochondriacs':
The gender pain gap

Recent years have also seen a growing number of conversations emerge around what's been dubbed the 'gender pain gap'. The term describes a long-established gender discrepancy in the way men and women experience pain, and the way in which their pain is treated. However, these conversations – at least in mainstream media – have typically centred on female-specific issues like the menstrual pain we explored in chapter 2 and vaginal pain (see chapter 6). In reality, the gender pain gap is much broader, impacting on the care that all women in pain receive, even when that pain relates to a condition or body part that's ostensibly gender-neutral.

Perhaps the most influential research in this area is 'The girl who cried pain: A bias against women in the treatment of pain', an article written by professors Diane Hoffmann and Anita Tarzian and published in the *Journal of Law, Medicine and Ethics* in 2001. 'The girl who cried pain' explores the role of biological, psychological and cultural gender differences in the way men and women experience pain, as well as the impact of gender bias on treatment.

'Research indicates that differences between men and women exist in the experience of pain, with women experiencing and reporting both more frequent and greater pain. Yet rather than receiving greater or at least as effective treatment for their pain as men, women are more likely to be less well treated than men for their painful symptoms,' the paper concludes. 'There are numerous factors that contribute to this undertreatment, but the literature supports the conclusion that there are gender-based biases regarding women's pain experiences.'

Specifically, Hoffmann and Tarzian say women's self-reports of pain are discounted, at least until there is objective evidence for the cause of their pain. This focus on objective factors, as well as cultural gender stereotypes, leaves women at greater risk of inadequate pain relief and continued suffering. Hoffmann and Tarzian's recommendations included improving medical education and ensuring women's voices are heard, but in the 20 years since 'The girl who cried pain' was published, depressingly little has changed.

More recent studies have found that women in pain are kept waiting longer in A&E than men; are less likely to be taken seriously; less likely to be prescribed opioid painkillers; and more likely to be prescribed sedatives or anti-anxiety medication. Anecdotally too, women in both acute and chronic pain tell me about being dismissed as 'anxious', 'hysterical', 'attention-seeking' and 'hypochondriacs'. These gender disparities are amplified by race and other intersecting biases, with Black patients half as likely to receive pain medication as white patients. The 2016 US study I mentioned in chapter 1 found that 50% of white medical students and postgraduate trainees held at least one false belief about biological differences between races, including 'Black people's skin is thicker than white people's skin' and 'Black people's nerve endings are less sensitive than white people's'. Crucially, those who held these false beliefs also showed racial bias in how much pain they perceived patients as experiencing and the treatment recommendations they made.

Among LGBTQ+ patients, research by Stonewall shows that lesbian women, trans and non-binary patients – as well as disabled LGBTQ+ people and Black, Asian and minority ethnic

LGBTQ+ people – were the most likely to experience unequal treatment, inappropriate curiosity and a lack of understanding from healthcare professionals. Disabled women, trans men and non-binary people, including those living with chronic illnesses, mental health issues or learning disabilities, also face additional barriers, which I'll explore further in chapters 4 and 5.

It's worth pointing out that much, if not all, of the research into the gender pain gap has focused on gender differences between cis men and cis women. Much less well researched is where trans patients fit into all this. 'The girl who cried pain', for example, highlights that reproductive hormones 'appear to influence sex-based pain differences.' There is also research suggesting that 'marked changes in sex hormones [i.e. through gender-affirming hormone therapy] affect the occurrence of pain' in some, but not all, trans patients. However, there is much that is still not well understood about the biological similarities and differences between trans men and women, and their cis peers, and how these are affected by the extent of someone's gender-affirming treatments.

What we do know is that trans women and 'feminine'-presenting non-binary people are subject to many of the same gender biases as cis women, and – as we'll explore later in this chapter – all trans and non-binary people are also subject to anti-trans biases, leading to health inequalities and treatment barriers of their own. Indeed, when it comes to acute illness and injury, your best chance of prompt and effective treatment is to be a cis man – preferably white, able-bodied, straight, middle class and with a 'healthy' BMI.

'Medical misogyny is ingrained in our training as doctors. We are actually taught that if a working age man comes to see their GP, you ought to sit up and take note because working age men do not see their GPs,' says former GP Dr Emma Reinhold. 'It's therefore ingrained in us to think much more deeply if a 29-year-old man comes through the door, for example, than if a 29-year-old woman comes through the door. There's perceived to be a much higher threshold for a man to come to the doctor, whereas women are just worried in general and come to the doctors all the time.'

This perception isn't necessarily backed up by the facts. Different studies have reached conflicting conclusions on this, but one found that: 'Given the strength of assumptions that women consult more readily for common symptoms, the evidence… was surprisingly weak and inconsistent.' Nevertheless, the gender bias persists – and it can be fatal.

*

One of the starkest examples of this bias in action is the 'heart attack gender gap'. Research, published as part of the 2019 *Bias and Biology* report by the British Heart Foundation (BHF), found gender disparities at every stage of heart attack care, from diagnosis to treatment and aftercare. As a result, the report estimates, more than 8000 women in England and Wales died needlessly from heart attacks over a 10-year period, purely because they'd received worse quality care than men.

Lorraine Kinzel, who I interviewed when the report came out, suffered a heart attack at just 44 years old. Her symptoms were initially misdiagnosed as a hiatus hernia and Lorraine waited in A&E for two hours before anyone realised she was actually having a heart attack. This isn't unusual; the *Bias and Biology* research shows that women are 50% more likely than men to receive an incorrect initial diagnosis when having a heart attack, and previous research found that women are seven times more likely than men to be misdiagnosed and discharged in the middle of a heart attack.

After being fitted with a stent, doctors reassured Lorraine that she was young and would bounce back, before discharging her from hospital with no aftercare or cardiac rehabilitation. Within five weeks, though, she was suffering from pain and breathlessness – symptoms of angina. Despite her history, doctors dismissed these symptoms as anxiety and panic attacks.

It took seven months of being sent away in pain before Lorraine was finally granted the angiogram she'd been pleading for. Lo and behold, it showed another arterial blockage and a second stent was fitted. Describing one particularly patronising cardiologist – who'd patted Lorraine on the shoulder, told her she was fine and her symptoms were 'just muscular' – she said, 'I felt so angry, like he thought I was a ditzy woman who didn't know what symptoms I was having.'

The BHF research is particularly shocking, but the gender gap highlighted by *Bias and Biology* was not a new discovery. More than 30 years ago, in 1991, cardiologist Dr Bernadine Healy coined the term 'Yentl Syndrome' to describe the different ways men and women are treated after heart attacks. (Yentl, heroine of an Isaac Bashevis Singer short story and a Barbra Streisand film, disguised herself as a man in order to get an education). For a long time this was blamed on sex differences in the way men and women's heart attack symptoms present. The belief was that male symptoms were seen as the 'default', while women's 'atypical' symptoms were often missed by medics. However, more recent research has shown this is largely a myth.

Although there are some sex differences in symptom presentation, research suggests these are 'modest'. In fact, according to one paper published in 2019, women are *more* likely than men to experience 'typical' symptoms. This research, published in the *Journal of the American Heart Association*, found the most common indicator of a heart attack was chest pain, which was the primary symptom for 91% of men and 92% of women. Women were also more likely than men to report other classic heart attack symptoms, including palpitations, nausea and pain radiating to their left arm, back, neck or jaw. Incorrect beliefs and assumptions about 'atypical' or 'female' heart attack symptoms could, therefore, actually put women at greater risk of underdiagnosis and treatment.

While differences in symptom presentation may previously have been overstated, the BHF's *Bias and Biology* report describes the heart attack gender gap as a 'deeply entrenched issue', likely caused by a complex combination of biological differences and gender bias. 'We know that women have slightly smaller hearts and their coronary arteries are slightly smaller. There's a tendency for women to less frequently have blocked coronary arteries and, when they do, those blockages are much smaller and further down the arteries, which can be harder to treat,' Professor Chris Gale, a professor of cardiovascular medicine at the University of Leeds, told me. Women's historic exclusion from medical research also contributes to the issue, he added, as well as unconscious gender bias and the widespread misconception that heart attacks only affect middle-aged men.

Again, this kind of bias is deeply embedded in the medical school curriculum. Writing for the BMA's journal, the *BMJ*, medical student Marina Politis says, 'Medical education might have you believe that as future doctors we will solely be treating men. Whether it is an anatomical model, textbook or multiple-choice question, our teaching resources are often centred on a male norm as the default.' She cites examples like, 'Mr X presents with central crushing chest pain,' and points out: 'A quick Google search on how to place the leads for an electrocardiogram reveals endless versions of the same chest, but none dare feature a breast. If I open any clinical examination textbook in the library, after flipping to the cardiology chapter, it too confronts me almost exclusively with male bodies.'

In reality, coronary heart disease, which causes most heart attacks, is the leading cause of death for women globally, killing twice as many women in the UK as breast cancer. Another study, published in 2021, found that 'non-traditional risk factors' for both heart attack and stroke, including work-related stress, sleep disorders and fatigue, are rising more steeply in women than men. Female heart attacks are not rare and, while there may be some sex differences, these aren't significant enough to account for the kind of diagnosis, treatment and aftercare gap that currently exists. Quite simply, doctors should be able to identify and treat heart attacks in women just as well as they would in a man.

However, there's also a broader cultural awareness issue. Pervasive media images of the 'Hollywood heart attack', where a silver-haired man clutches his chest in pain before falling to the ground, may result in women, as well as their doctors, being slower to recognise the symptoms in themselves. When having a heart attack, research shows women are typically slower to go to hospital than men, often because they dismiss their own symptoms or don't connect the dots. Combine that with the fact that women are more likely to be misdiagnosed once they arrive in hospital and you've got a potentially deadly double whammy of treatment delays.

*

A&E departments play a hugely important role when it comes to diagnosing the causes of acute pain, as well as triaging and treating, or referring on to specialists. In many ways this puts A&E doctors in a similar position to GPs. While frustrated patients may see them as the treatment gatekeepers, they also face enormous practical challenges themselves, from waiting time pressures to the same under-resourcing issues we've already discussed. But, as the research shows, doctors in emergency medicine are certainly not immune from bias either. They do make mistakes, they do get it wrong – and the consequences can be huge.

Queer, biracial student Rhian Arnold was just 20 when she presented to A&E, having found herself suddenly struck down by excruciating back pain and breathing difficulties. There she was eventually given an X-ray and some co-codamol, told her symptoms were 'just back pain', and instructed to go home and rest. 'The tone of hospital staff was sharp. Almost degrading. I felt guilty, like I'd wasted their time,' she writes. The next day, though, she was back, after staff at college called an ambulance. 'I was screaming uncontrollably and unable to move. In A&E, after hours of being ignored while I drifted in and out of consciousness, I was again told there was nothing wrong with me,' Rhian says. She was given diazepam – an anti-anxiety medication, which knocked her out – and told not to come back, as she was wasting her own time and theirs.

By day three, Rhian says, everything went by in a blur. Her mum had travelled down to London from the Midlands to look after her and, when Rhian again ended up being rushed into A&E with excruciating pain and breathing difficulties, it was her mum who refused to take no for an answer. As a result of her mum's strong will, Rhian was diagnosed with pneumonia, pleurisy, pleural empyema, a flooded chest cavity and an almost fully collapsed lung – a combination that would likely be fatal for anyone elderly or vulnerable, but which is virtually unheard of in an otherwise healthy woman of Rhian's age.

'Talks were had about what would happen if I didn't make it and a meeting was held with my year group at college about how I may not return,' she says. 'Two weeks and a million injections, blood tests, IV lines, antibiotics and a chest drain later, I was allowed to go home to start rebuilding my life, which turned out to be the biggest task yet.' Rhian's relationship with her then girlfriend and family suffered as a result of the trauma, and she describes experiencing horrifying flashbacks of what she'd been through. 'My local hospital had simply brushed me off as a young girl "wasting their time" and had let me get just hours away from death,' she says.

Of course, the severity of Rhian's illness is extremely rare. Most young women turned away from hospital with an eye-roll and a diazepam don't find themselves at death's door within 24 hours. But, depressingly, the attitudes that she encountered are still far less rare. Perhaps most striking – and it's a story that you'll hear again and again throughout this book – is the over reliance on one single diagnostic test at the expense of the patient's self-reported symptoms. When an X-ray showed no objective evidence of a problem, her obvious pain, distress and inability to breathe were so easily written off. While the doctors she encountered in A&E can perhaps be forgiven for not realising quite how critical Rhian's condition was, their outright dismissal of her very apparent pain and distress is much harder to stomach.

Even two years on, Rhian says she still experiences flashbacks and emotional breakdowns, but counts her lucky stars that she's still here and thriving. 'I will always have pain in my left side and who knows how it will affect me in later life. The mental scars may never fully heal, but I do like to think of it as a reminder that I'm a survivor,' she says. 'The fact that doctors are still pityingly shaking their heads at young women, telling them they're fine and don't know what they're talking about, fills me with rage. But, by sharing my story, I hope to raise awareness and inspire young women to stand up for themselves.'

*

Besides gender, sexuality, race and age, weight stigma is another significant barrier when it comes to accessing healthcare – and studies have repeatedly shown that this form of bias disproportionately affects women. Former NHS GP Dr Asher Larmie, who is non-binary and blogs as The Fat Doctor, says fatphobia is rife in the medical profession and is something they spent many years internalising themself.

'Doctors almost universally hold some kind of anti-fat bias. A study on 4732 medical students showed that two-thirds of them had conscious, explicit, anti-fat bias and three-quarters had implicit bias,' they say. 'Studies show that doctors are less inclined to examine fat patients, and often doctors will blame the patient's weight rather than looking for a diagnosis. So instead of saying, "I'm going to start you on this treatment" or "I'm going to refer you for surgery," they say, "You need to lose some weight and your symptoms will get better." That massively impacts patients' care and has been shown to lead to delayed treatment.'

In one study, 84% of patients in larger bodies reported that their weight is blamed for most medical problems. Not only can this weight stigma cause significant harm, it also relies on an unreliable metric, body mass index (BMI), which is in itself inherently biased. BMI is based on height/weight ratios in white, European men and was never designed to be used as a measure of individual health – yet that is exactly how it is used today. A systematic review found that BMI only has a one in three success rate when it comes to accurately predicting cardiometabolic health, meaning you cannot accurately identify how healthy or otherwise someone is based purely on their BMI. For women and ethnic minorities, the fact that it's based on white male data means it's an even less reliable measure.

Despite this, the health service seems wedded to BMI and the diagnosis of 'obesity', including as a way of rationing services. According to a 2016 report by the Royal College of Surgeons (RCS), patients who are overweight, as well as those who smoke, are treated as 'soft targets' for NHS savings. The report looked at routine, non-urgent surgeries and found that almost a third of NHS clinical commissioning groups, which make the decisions about NHS services in the areas of England that they serve, had at least one policy restricting access to treatments based on BMI. This, it states, is 'in contravention of national clinical guidance' and such blanket bans 'do not best serve patient care.'

Three women I interviewed in 2020 had all been told to lose weight before undergoing treatment, respectively for gallstones, fertility problems and endometriosis. Two of these women found themselves pushed into restrictive 'quick fix' diets that were unhealthy, unsustainable and not clinically necessary, and all three were left distressed and suffering in the meantime.

As a consequence of this kind of treatment, Asher adds, weight stigma also directly harms fatter patients' faith in the medical system, making them less likely to seek healthcare in future. 'Patients who are stigmatised by their doctor because of their weight are less likely to trust their doctor and less likely to go back,' they explain. In one study, 68% of women with high BMIs reported that they delayed seeking healthcare because of their weight and 83% said their weight was a barrier to getting appropriate healthcare.

'As a 40-year-old who was assigned female at birth and has been a GP since 2009, I have certainly been avoiding my own GP for years, because I'm afraid of being stigmatised again,' Asher says. 'Women say things to me like, "I've got a breast lump, but I don't want to see my doctor because I'm scared they're going to shame me." That terrifies me, because all it's going to do is cause more deaths and more poor health.'

Similarly, by the time ly h Kerr's symptoms started, she had already internalised the message that being fat is automatically unhealthy. 'I accepted the consensus that fat was bad and thin was good. I was in the process of some seriously unhealthy dieting when I initially experienced quite serious gastric pain. There were other symptoms, vomiting and difficulty eating, but pain was the standout,' she writes.

When she progressed from short bursts to hour-long stints of excruciating pain, ly saw her GP, who said it was most likely indigestion and/or heartburn. These could be surprisingly painful, she was assured, but if she changed her diet and lost some weight, things would improve. 'I tightened up my already drastic diet and continued to lose weight. My symptoms did not improve. In fact, they worsened,' ly says. She began to have 'torturous' prolonged periods of pain, lasting for days at a time, during which she was unable to eat, move or sleep.

During repeated visits to A&E though, ly was again told she had indigestion or heartburn and advised to lose weight. 'No one listened when I told them I was barely eating. No one cared that I was losing lots of weight. All the doctors were dismissive of my pain. Most were patronising. Some were hostile. No one helped,' she says.

After more than a year of this, ly recalls one particularly traumatic visit to A&E, during which she was throwing up blood and bile, and in so much pain she could barely speak. 'I saw a deeply unpleasant man who vacillated between [viewing me as] a hysterical woman [or] an addict seeking drugs. He gave me a cup of peptac, an antacid, which I promptly threw up, and sent me home,' she says. 'I felt utterly beaten that night. I knew there was something wrong with me. There was no way I could feel this bad and there not be a problem. But no one would listen. I was tired of being judged and looked down upon. I went home, lay down and cried.'

Like Rhian, it was the advocacy of ly's mother that eventually got her a diagnosis – and just in time, too. 'My mum was shocked when she saw the state I was in and insisted we return to A&E. With someone fighting fit to advocate for me I was finally taken seriously. A doctor ordered the simple blood test that would diagnose me with pancreatitis,' she says. 'By the time those bloods had come back, my body had gone into shock. Had I not returned to hospital that night, I would have likely died – all because medical professionals wouldn't look past the size of my belly.'

ly spent the next seven days in the high dependency unit (HDU). She was catheterised, fed fluids via an IV drip and given a morphine pump. She doesn't even remember that first week in hospital. What she did learn later was that although she didn't fit the usual profile for pancreatitis (typically older men, big meat eaters and heavy drinkers), she did have classic symptoms. 'The pain I'd been describing was textbook. The onset and progression of symptoms was exactly what was to be expected of pancreatitis. Had someone taken a minute to listen to me, I could have been diagnosed on my first trip to A&E,' ly says. 'I really believe, if I hadn't been a fat woman, that's probably what would have happened.'

After several more bouts of pancreatitis, as well as gallbladder issues, ly discovered her weight wasn't even the problem. 'The most likely culprit was spending my 20s yo-yo dieting. The fad dieting and resultant weight loss that doctors had always encouraged actually made me ill,' she says.

This type of harm, Asher says, is also well-established and is something they frequently see in patients suffering digestive issues like pancreatitis and gallstones. However, they add, the evidence is too often overlooked by a medical profession which, like the rest of society, is obsessed with eradicating fatness at any cost. 'Rapid weight loss has also been shown to cause issues like gallstones and if you lose more than 15% of your body weight that actually reduces your life expectancy quite significantly,' they explain.

Meanwhile, Asher adds, our cultural obsession with dieting has many people – particularly women, who encounter the most pressure to lose weight – trapped in a miserable and unhealthy vicious cycle. 'The more people diet and fixate on losing weight, the more likely they are to gain weight in the long term and the more likely they are to develop disordered eating. Encouraging people to go on diets is actually fuelling the so-called obesity epidemic. Not only is it not healthy, it's actively making things worse,' they explain.

A 2021 report by the Women and Equalities Committee recommended ditching the health service's counterproductive obsession with BMI and instead adopting a 'Health At Every Size' (HAES) approach. HAES is a weight inclusive health movement for which Asher also advocates. It's based on the principles of respect and body diversity; challenging scientific and cultural assumptions; valuing lived experiences; and encouraging compassionate self-care through joyful and intuitive movement and eating.

'The Health At Every Size movement is treated like a joke; nobody takes it seriously, even though it's well established and based on really good evidence. Instead, we have smoke and mirrors. The government wants to be seen to be doing something, like putting calories on restaurant menus, even though the evidence shows this does more harm than good,' Asher says.

Determined to address medicine's fatphobia from inside the profession, Asher is currently collecting patient stories, and organising training on weight stigma for healthcare professionals and the public. 'Education is massively important and the more stories and experiences we collect, the more damning the evidence is,' they explain. In addition, Asher would like to see the government conduct an inquiry into weight stigma, and for the General Medical Council (GMC) to regulate against it. 'They have a responsibility to prove their doctors are not discriminating against patients,' they say.

★

When it comes to navigating a discriminatory healthcare system, trans and non-binary patients are subject to many of the same biases as their cis female peers. Their symptoms may be put down to their weight, their mental health history or assumed anxiety, or downplayed on the basis of their race or their (actual or perceived) gender. But they also face a phenomenon known colloquially as 'trans broken arm syndrome', a term coined to describe when healthcare professionals put even the most routine of symptoms (tonsillitis, a broken arm, mental health difficulties and so on) down to their patient's trans status or hormone treatments.

As a result of this, trans patients may be denied treatment altogether, on the basis that the healthcare professional in front of them 'doesn't know how to deal with trans people' or they may find themselves referred back to gender identity services for an issue that's entirely unrelated to their transition.

Transition-specific healthcare is itself notoriously fraught with issues. In 2015, independent watchdog Healthwatch said the NHS 'treats trans patients as second-class citizens' and warned that delays to treatment were leading to patients considering self-harm and suicide. Today the situation is even worse, with years-long waiting lists just for an initial gender identity services appointment.

After this, many trans patients face an 'intrusive and degrading' assessment process of 'proving' their gender before they can begin their transition. Some doctors are even still telling trans women they aren't wearing enough lipstick or 'feminine' clothing, according to evidence given to the Women and

Equalities Select Committee in 2021. Conforming to these kinds of outdated gender stereotypes is not officially a requirement of the process, but many trans people feel under pressure to present themselves in this way because they're scared that not doing so might risk a clinician seeing them as 'not trans enough'.

While these issues are largely beyond the scope of this book, they do provide important context to the issues trans people face in other, more general areas of healthcare. They also sit alongside a broader, and increasingly vicious, societal transphobia, which inevitably impacts on the way trans patients are received by healthcare professionals. During the course of researching this book, I've heard about healthcare professionals whose behaviour towards their trans patients ranged from supportive but ignorant to downright abusive.

Stonewall's 2018 report on LGBTQ+ healthcare in the UK found that a third of trans people have experienced some form of unequal treatment from healthcare staff because of their trans status, and 20% had witnessed discriminatory or negative remarks by healthcare staff in the previous year. Half of trans people and a third of non-binary people said they'd experienced inappropriate curiosity, and one in four trans patients had been outed by healthcare professionals without their consent, either in front of other staff or other patients.

More recently, in a 2021 survey by trans-led advocacy group TransActual, 70% of respondents said they'd experienced some form of transphobia while accessing general (not transition-related) healthcare, 14% reported they'd been refused GP care on at least one occasion because they were trans and 57% said they avoided going to the doctors when they were unwell.

One trans woman, Marie, tells me about going to A&E with kidney stones, 'one of the most painful things you can imagine,' more than a decade after transitioning. After discussions about her medication revealed Marie was trans and taking oestrogen, her doctor responded: 'Ah, this is probably why you have the kidney stones. Hormones are not sweeties!' While research (carried out in post-menopausal cis women on HRT) does show an increased risk of kidney stones for women on oestrogen, Marie had been taking the minimum possible dose for years.

Regardless of her personal risk level, there is something so patronising, so minimising in this doctor's words – a subtly transphobic implication that Marie's gender-affirming treatment is some kind of frivolous, needlessly hazardous indulgence. Yet the reality for many trans people is that these treatments are lifesaving. Marie's kidney stones were eventually treated, 'but only after they'd made me think [it] was my own fault,' she adds.

Concerns about the use of hormones were a common theme in many of the stories I heard. Several women have told me about doctors blaming oestrogen for their long-term skin conditions, despite them having started on hormone treatment much more recently. One of them, Cassie, says, 'I've had chronic skin conditions, including eczema, all my life and recently a new GP at my practice tried to blame it on HRT, which I've only been on for six years. It's maddening. I have next to no faith in doctors anymore since transitioning.'

Meanwhile, trans man Jack (not his real name) tells me he was initially refused antibiotics after a nasty cut on his hand got infected. This, he was told, was because, 'They needed to check whether it would work with testosterone – which isn't something they'd do before prescribing standard antibiotics to a cis guy.' It was only after speaking with Jack's gender specialist that his GP, three days later, agreed to write a prescription for the antibiotics. 'Fortunately, it didn't get much worse while I was waiting, but three days waiting for antibiotics when you've got an infection could be the difference between it being treatable at home and needing hospitalisation,' Jack says.

After her transition, Alice was denied a routine blood test by two GPs in her surgery, with one of them – who had treated her for 10 years before she came out as trans – saying, 'I'm not comfortable treating transgender people.' When she contacted a different surgery, the GP she spoke to told her he was 'not against transgender people, he just didn't know how to treat us.' Eventually, after contacting three alternative practices, Alice found a surgery where the 'absolutely brilliant' GP booked her in for the blood test without so much as batting an eyelid.

Clearly the contrast between these approaches demonstrates that GPs do have the capacity to treat trans patients if they're so inclined. This is beautifully illustrated by the experience that trans woman Josi shared with me: 'Some years ago, having socially transitioned, I approached my GP for help. She said, "I'm totally ignorant with no experience of transgender issues. Come back next week, I will find out and help." She kept to her word and the whole practice is an exemplar of [how it should be done],' she says. Too often though, a lack of confidence, confusion, or just straight-up prejudice can all leave trans people facing needless barriers to basic, straightforward healthcare.

My friend Harry (not his real name), for example, describes huge difficulties finding a local doctor or nurse to remove his catheter following gender-affirming lower surgery. 'I had written instructions from my consultant and specialist nurses, which explained that it was just like any other catheter, but I had to beg and plead to find a medical professional who was willing to provide this simple and necessary care,' he says. 'I was in a lot of pain, and physically and emotionally really vulnerable, but they were trying to send me all the way back to London [to my surgical team] for something which takes 30 seconds and which any doctor or nurse should be able to do.'

After a GP eventually agreed to remove the catheter, Harry recalls one nurse – who had previously refused to help – choosing to loiter inside the curtain, 'to get an eyeful of my fascinating genitals while the doctor removed it.' This whole experience had a profound impact on him. 'Being looked at and spoken to in this way when I was so vulnerable changed the way I feel about being trans "in the world" and made me a more guarded and cynical person. After years of being very open and vocal about my transition, I'm now only out to family and close friends,' Harry says.

Other examples, shared on the hashtag #TransDocFail, include being denied care for a heart condition, 'because I have all this gender stuff going on, so it was probably in my head'; an A&E doctor's insistence on carrying out a genital examination before doing an X-ray for chest pain; and 'having my physical condition repeatedly dismissed as psychosomatic because I'm trans and also have [mental health] problems.'

Perhaps unsurprisingly, one study found that nearly 50% of trans and gender non-conforming patients avoid going to the emergency department when they need acute care, citing fear of discrimination, length of wait and negative previous experiences as their reasons. Many of the issues discussed here are unique to trans patients – from the refusal to carry out routine, gender-neutral procedures like taking blood from someone's arm, to the intrusive, inappropriate curiosity about people's genitals. However, they also have a lot in common with the issues cis women face.

'There are so many parallels with misogyny in medicine, so trans people have a very natural allegiance with feminist positions on things like agency around reproductive capacity,' says Dr Ben Vincent, a non-binary academic and author of *Transgender Health: A Practitioner's Guide to Binary and Non-Binary Trans Patient Care*. 'You hear of [trans patients] being refused hysterectomies or breast reductions on the basis of things like, "What are your husband's thoughts on this?" It's the same logic which underpins the idea that you don't get to make the decision, because it rubs up against expectations of gendered bodies in our society,' they say.

Ben believes healthcare professionals refusing to treat trans patients largely comes down to ignorance and fear. 'Sometimes doctors will say something is complex when in reality it's just that they don't know how easy it is; they're using "complexity" as a bit of a get out clause,' they explain. Other times, Ben adds, 'We just have a really dramatic lack of evidence, which comes from a failure to accommodate trans people [in research], just like there's been a failure to accommodate cis women.'

YOUR PHYSICAL HEALTH AND PAIN TOOLKIT

This chapter has been something of a whistle-stop tour, cramming in just a few of the myriad gender-neutral physical health issues that anyone may face over the course of a lifetime. As we've seen, though, cis women, trans and non-binary patients face a whole range of intersecting barriers to accessing acute or emergency care – with gendered biases exacerbated by discrimination on the grounds of race, class, weight, sexuality, mental health history or trans status.

We've known for a long time that the gender pain gap exists, but it isn't going anywhere fast and all these prejudices remain very deeply embedded within the medical system. So much of this needs a radical change from the inside out, beginning with a re-education of doctors about the conscious and unconscious biases that may impact their care. For healthcare professionals working under stressful, highly pressurised conditions in A&E, for example, decisions about who to prioritise must be made quickly – but this pressure can easily result in falling back on lazy stereotypes and biases, which almost never serve the most marginalised patients in the waiting room.

For patients, perhaps the most useful tip for accessing acute or emergency care is to take an advocate with you if possible. Particularly when you're in significant pain and distress, having someone who can speak up on your behalf can be invaluable or, at the very least, provides a witness to the treatment you've received. Even if this isn't possible, it's important to be aware of the signs and symptoms of health emergencies like heart attacks, as well as any relevant family history or personal risk factors you may have. Trust your gut when you know something is wrong and seek help at the earliest possible opportunity.

Try to describe your pain or symptoms clearly, in as much detail as possible. Is it a sharp, stabbing pain or a dull ache? Where exactly in your body is affected? Do you have other symptoms? Exactly how long has this been going on? What impact is it having on your everyday life? If possible, it may also be worth looking up possible causes for your symptoms, so you can ask your doctor: 'Could it be X? Is there a test you can do?' or 'Can you explain why you don't think it's Y?'

As I've said before, though, remember that it's not your fault if your own advocacy, or the advocacy of whoever's accompanying you, doesn't get results. Research published in 2020 found that: 'Women scored higher than men on measures of patient likelihood to self-advocate. Women also reported intending to use more varied self-advocacy strategies than men. This suggests it is unlikely that patients' communication styles are to blame for the gender pain gap.' If you do need extra backup, every NHS hospital has a Patient Advice and Liaison Service (PALS), which you can contact for advice and support. You're also entitled to make a complaint and PALS can provide information on how to do so.

If you've been dismissed or denied treatment based on your weight, Dr Asher Larmie recommends checking out the HAES Health Sheets website (listed below). This site contains a range of self-advocacy resources, research and 'blame-free, shame-free' information on a variety of health issues, including heart disease, PCOS and type 2 diabetes.

For trans and non-binary people, TransActual offers a comprehensive range of information on transition-specific and general trans healthcare, with resources for both healthcare professionals and patients.

Resources
- British Heart Foundation – bhf.org.uk
- British Lung Foundation – blf.org.uk
- Fat Doctor UK – fatdoctor.co.uk
- Guts UK – gutscharity.org.uk
- HAES Health Sheets – haeshealthsheets.com
- Stroke Association – stroke.org.uk
- TransActual – transactual.org.uk/healthcare

4

'Chronically female': Why disability is a feminist issue

In the previous chapter I focused on acute pain, illness and injury, but the gender health gap undoubtedly also extends to chronic and disabling conditions. While women's slightly longer life expectancy is sometimes cited (by men) as proof that gender inequality doesn't exist, it's worth noting that this 'mortality advantage' is offset by the fact that women spend more of their lives with poor health and disability.

The term 'disability' covers a broad range of conditions and is, in and of itself, fairly gender-neutral. There's absolutely no doubt that disabled people of all genders are disadvantaged by our ableist and inaccessible world. However, data published by the UK Government for the year 2018/19 shows that disability is more prevalent in women (7.7 million) than men (6.3 million).

Chronic pain is one of the leading causes of disability worldwide, affecting more than a third of the UK population. It's also, as you may have guessed, more common in women than in men. According to the International Association for the Study of Pain, 'Chronic pain affects a higher proportion of women than men around the world; however, women are less likely to receive treatment. Research has shown that women generally experience more recurrent pain, more severe pain and longer-lasting pain than men.'

Among the chronic pain conditions that disproportionately affect women are fibromyalgia (of which 80–90% of diagnosed cases are women), IBS, rheumatoid arthritis, osteoarthritis, temporomandibular joint disorder (TMJ), chronic pelvic pain and migraine headaches. Then, of course, there are chronic pain conditions specific to those assigned female at birth, like endometriosis and vulvodynia.

As always, this is an intersectional issue, with gender just one factor implicated in the prevalence of chronic pain. The *Unseen, Unequal, Unfair* report into chronic pain in England, published in 2021 by charity Versus Arthritis, highlights that chronic pain is more prevalent in areas of greater deprivation. In England's most deprived areas, 45% of women and 37% of men report chronic pain, compared to 33% of women and 27% of men in less deprived areas.

There is also, the report highlights, 'an increased burden of chronic pain on people from some minority ethnic backgrounds'. Chronic pain affects 44% of Black people, 35% of Asian people, 34% of mixed-race people and 34% of white people, with those from Asian backgrounds most likely to report experiencing 'high impact pain'.

Women make up almost 80% of those affected by autoimmune diseases, which include rheumatoid arthritis, multiple sclerosis (MS) and lupus. They are disproportionately affected by chronic, multi-system disorders like myalgic encephalomyelitis (ME, also controversially known as chronic fatigue syndrome or ME/CFS), postural orthostatic tachycardia syndrome (PoTS), Ehlers-Danlos syndrome (EDS) and mast cell activation syndrome (MCAS). And women also appear to be most affected by the emerging condition, or group of conditions, Long Covid.

What do all these conditions have in common, besides their prevalence in women? They're also chronically underfunded, under-researched and poorly understood. Some, like ME and fibromyalgia, have also long been 'contested illnesses', with some doctors disputing their existence altogether. Patients with these conditions frequently find themselves disbelieved by doctors, their symptoms dismissed as 'psychosomatic' and the conditions themselves wrongly written off as having no biological basis. Meanwhile, 62% of people with autoimmune diseases are labelled 'chronic complainers'.

While most of the gender data on prevalence of these conditions is based on cis women and cis men, it's notable that trans and non-binary patients also appear to be disproportionately affected by chronic illness and disability. Although research on this is even more scarce, one study noted higher burdens of disability in trans people than cis people. In particular, it found that 'gender-nonconforming people had higher odds of multiple chronic conditions, poor quality of life, and disabilities than both cisgender males and females.'

It's not clear why this is and a review of the evidence around chronic disease in transgender populations highlighted 'critical gaps in the existing transgender health literature landscape'. This gaping hole in chronic illness research is yet another example of the common ground that disabled cis women, trans and non-binary people share. If cis men were affected to the same extent by these same long-term, disabling conditions, would there be such a dearth of research? I personally suspect not.

As it stands, the knock-on effect for many patients living with chronic illness is that there's simply not enough known about their condition. In both research and medical training, long-term health issues that predominantly affect women are not prioritised. Consequently, as we'll explore, their symptoms are frequently dismissed as 'medically unexplained' or 'all in your head' and, even after diagnosis, there is often a serious lack of effective treatment and support available.

This isn't necessarily to say that cis men living with chronic illnesses have an easy time of it. They too share the frustrations of having conditions that are poorly understood by the medical establishment and some may face the additional stigma of living with a 'feminised' illness. However, among chronic pain patients, research suggests men's symptoms are generally better managed by healthcare professionals – with women receiving 'less adequate pain medication and more antidepressants compared to men'.

One literature review concluded that: 'Compared to men, women have more pain, it is more accepted for women to show pain and more women are diagnosed with chronic pain syndromes. Yet, paradoxically, women's pain reports are taken less seriously, their pain is discounted as being psychic or non-existent, and their medication is less adequate than treatment given to men. This has been described as a paradox, but can be explained as an expression of hegemonic masculinity and andronormativity in health care.' In other words, women and other marginalised genders still find themselves at the bottom of the heap, precisely because men continue to be seen, and prioritised, as the medical default.

*

Among the 7.7 million disabled women in the UK, experiences of disability will vary – from lifelong physical or learning disabilities to those acquired later in life, either through injury or long-term illness. Despite this range of experiences, though, disabled women and gender minorities face several common challenges when it comes to accessing healthcare, from issues with accessibility through to ableist attitudes about their health and even the value of their lives.

'People are always surprised when I say the most ableism I ever get is at the doctor's, but there's this attitude that "I need to fix you but I can't, and therefore I don't want to know,"' says journalist and wheelchair user Lucy Webster, who has cerebral palsy – a lifelong condition affecting movement and coordination – as a result of medical negligence during her birth.

This view of disability as an 'unfixable' medical problem is not uncommon and it can have a significant impact on all other aspects of a disabled patient's health. Lucy, for example, recalls doctors dismissing other health problems – like significant, long-term insomnia – as simply part of her condition, rather than providing appropriate treatments and support.

Often, it seems, healthcare professionals are unable to look past Lucy's disability; unable to recognise that this sociable, professional, millennial woman might require adaptations to manage in her career and social life, or that she's just as likely as any other patient to need other, more general physical, mental and sexual healthcare. Instead, in her medical encounters, Lucy has been left feeling defined by her disability, not taken seriously, or even ignored altogether by doctors who address her carer instead of speaking directly to Lucy herself.

As a result of these experiences, Lucy says, she very rarely goes to the doctors these days. 'When you're disabled, they speak to you like you're seven years old or stupid. I didn't trust the healthcare system much to begin with, because my condition was caused by a doctor making a mistake, but now I have no faith at all,' she tells me.

In some ways, though, Lucy adds, 'I feel lucky that I don't have a chronic illness. At least doctors tend to know what cerebral palsy is and what it does,' she explains. You don't have to look far within the disabled community to find stories of women living with chronic, often unexplained, symptoms, who are struggling to be heard, believed or understood by their doctors. Whatever their symptoms, and whatever the ultimate diagnosis, the same thread of disbelief, dismissiveness and denial runs through so many of these experiences.

In 2018, my friend Sarah Cope was one of the first contributors to write for Hysterical Women, sharing her long struggle to find an explanation for her chronic back pain. She describes 16 years of pain, of being dismissed and sent away still in pain; 16 years of trying every treatment available, several of them multiple times. She adds, 'And let's not even think about the thousands of pounds I have spent in the process.' At one point, she recalls, an NHS clinician referred her for a course of cognitive behavioural therapy (CBT – a form of psychological therapy), explaining as he did so: 'It's not quite like we're saying it's all in your head, but it is, basically.'

Sarah's is sadly a familiar story. The symptoms and the number of years spent waiting for a diagnosis vary, but the experiences of being dismissed, or arrogantly assured that physical symptoms are 'all in your head', are all too predictable and all too reminiscent of hysteria.

Today, the term 'medically unexplained symptoms' is used to describe much of what would once have been written off as hysteria. But, while the terminology has moved on, the underlying attitudes have, in many cases, continued to lag behind. Women like Sarah still find themselves butting up against the pervasive idea that, if medicine can't explain something, it must be psychological. In reality, of course, 'medically unexplained' invariably turns out simply to mean 'not yet diagnosed' – typically because of a failure to properly investigate or identify the underlying cause.

Retired assistant headteacher Jane Green was disbelieved by doctors for decades before eventually, in her 50s, being diagnosed with hypermobile Ehlers-Danlos Syndrome (hEDS) – a connective tissue disorder which explained why, since her teens, she'd regularly experienced pain, bloating, migraines and dislocations. Meanwhile, Sarah's 'medically unexplained symptoms' were eventually explained with a diagnosis of the autoimmune condition psoriatic arthritis and, crucially, she received a long-awaited treatment plan.

*

As we've seen elsewhere, there are two key issues at play when it comes to the treatment of chronically ill women – what *Doing Harm* author Maya Dusenbery terms the 'knowledge gap' and the 'trust gap'. Ignorance of complex and female-dominant conditions makes it less likely that a typical doctor will land on the correct diagnosis, particularly in the space of a 10-minute general practice appointment. The lack of objective testing methods for many of these conditions also makes diagnosis difficult. Standard blood and imaging tests may come back 'normal' simply because they're not looking for the right things, but, for a medical profession that's increasingly reliant on diagnostic testing, this can easily be misinterpreted as 'there's nothing wrong'.

Meanwhile, the persistent and deep-rooted belief that women and minorities can't be trusted to accurately self-report their experiences provides a convenient alibi for health professionals who find themselves stumped by tricky symptom presentations. Rather than admit they don't know, or acknowledge that medical science is fallible, limited and constantly evolving, the trust gap sees healthcare professionals instead shift the blame towards their patient.

It's particularly ill-considered when you think of some of the other conditions that, in the past, found themselves labelled as 'hysterical' or 'psychological'. Prior to the emergence of MRI technology, MS was one of the female-dominant conditions studied by Freud's predecessor, Jean-Martin Charcot, whose work lumped hysteria together with various neurological conditions and mental illnesses. Though MRI scans can now provide objective evidence of the condition, its association with hysteria still persists in the experiences of some MS patients. Writing for Hysterical Women, Hayley Crowther describes being made to feel like a 'time-waster' and a 'complete idiot' by one neurologist, who 'scoffed' and 'rolled her eyes at me', before MRI results proved she did, in fact, genuinely have the neurological condition.

Indeed, the 'psychologisation' of physical symptoms that we saw in the previous chapter is perhaps at its most pervasive when it comes to these feminised, difficult to diagnose long-term illnesses. Ellie Hopkins lives with multiple chronic conditions, and is the founder and CEO of Chronically Awesome, an online community and registered charity for patients with chronic illnesses. Writing for Hysterical Women in 2020, she described how women subject to this kind of psychologisation are effectively labelled 'hysterical until proven otherwise.'

It's a risk that weighs heavily on many of those living with chronic illnesses. 'Living with chronic pain is a battle, one that wears you down over time,' Ellie wrote. 'To make progress you have to become an expert in your body, your illness and the medical specialisms you fall under. You have to learn to advocate for yourself, to stand up to medical professionals, to fight for the treatment you want. It's hard. It's even harder – nearly impossible – if you feel like no one is on your side, fighting your corner, helping you navigate treatment pathways and decisions that could impact the rest of your life.'

While these are typically not the same life-or-death scenarios as a heart attack being dismissed as a panic attack, they nevertheless have a profound impact, not least on the mental wellbeing of those with chronic illnesses. In 2019 Chronically Awesome surveyed nearly 700 members on their experiences, of whom 94% were female. The majority lived with symptoms like fatigue, pain, dizziness or light headedness, migraines, reduced mobility and loss of strength; 95% of respondents also reported feeling lonely or isolated; while three-quarters said they experience depression and/or anxiety.

Despite this, 43% of respondents had avoided seeking help for emotional difficulties for fear of having their physical symptoms wrongly labelled as psychological – a fear that, as I'll explore in the next chapter, too often proves to be well-founded. Meanwhile, 41% of respondents had experienced PTSD as a result of their illness and/or their treatment.

A separate survey of almost 800 disabled women and non-binary people, carried out by Chronic Illness Inclusion in 2021, found that a third of respondents had waited more than 10 years for a diagnosis. Before receiving their current diagnosis, four out of five had their physical symptoms attributed to psychosocial causes – such as anxiety, stress or being overweight – and roughly half had received psychological therapy.

Hopefully it goes without saying that developing a life-altering, or even debilitating long-term condition at any point in your life would take a toll on anyone's mental health. Chronic pain, fatigue, inflammation and mobility issues inevitably come with significant changes to your everyday life, impacting on your career, family and romantic relationships, social life and more. The fact that most chronically ill patients do experience isolation, depression and anxiety is hardly surprising when you actually pause to consider the life-changing impact of getting sick and not getting better. That's before you even take into account the medical trauma that many patients describe, resulting from not being believed or taken seriously by the very people they expected to make them better.

From the outside then, it's abundantly clear to me that these emotional difficulties are not the cause of anyone's symptoms, but the (entirely understandable) effect of living with a chronic illness or disability. Yet, in my own work, women have told me – just as Chronically Awesome's research shows – that they avoid seeking help for depression and anxiety in case it leads doctors to invalidate their physical symptoms. Likewise, the Chronic Illness Inclusion research confirms what I've seen time and time again over the years: that 'disbelief is the overarching theme' for women seeking healthcare for chronic illnesses.

While it's true of a whole range of symptoms and conditions, I hear this particularly from women with ME, the long-term, fluctuating, multisystem condition affecting 250,000 people in the UK, an estimated 75–80% of whom are women. ME is a neurological disease, characterised by chronic fatigue and post-exertional malaise – where symptoms are triggered by mental or physical exertion or sensory overload – as well as pain, muscle weakness, cognitive difficulties and symptoms of the gastrointestinal, autonomic, endocrine and immune systems.

Among patients with ME, it's clear that the trust gap runs in both directions. 'I've lost trust in doctors over 14 years of not being believed or understood,' says Jessica Taylor-Bearman, whose memoirs *A Girl Behind Dark Glasses* and *A Girl In One Room* recount her experiences as a bedbound young woman with severe ME. 'There's no apology, no "I'm sorry we didn't get this," no acknowledgement of the fact they got it so wrong. That then becomes a trust issue. Whenever I go into hospital and a doctor comes in, even now, I'm absolutely terrified,' she tells me.

ME, like many other chronic conditions, has a long history of being written off by mainstream medicine as psychosomatic or delusional, and treated using psychological therapies like CBT. While this kind of talking therapy can be useful for some patients as a way of coping with the emotional impact of ME on their life and mental health, the way it's long been framed as a 'treatment' or 'cure' for the condition itself is clearly unhelpful. Even more controversial has been the use of graded exercise therapy (GET), a structured exercise programme that aims to gradually increase physical activity, but which actively harmed many patients with ME.

After a review of evidence proved they're ineffective at best and harmful at worst, both CBT and GET have now finally been removed from treatment guidelines for ME, with the caveat that CBT can still be offered to help patients manage their symptoms. In May 2022, at the launch of the All Party Parliamentary Group (APPG) on ME's 'Rethinking ME' report, then health secretary Sajid Javid promised 'radical action' for patients. As well as challenging the idea that ME is psychological, the government committed to funding more research into the condition, and providing better care and support for patients and their families.

Despite this progress, Jessica – and many more beside her – believe there's still a long way to go for ME patients to achieve the recognition and validation they deserve. 'Even though I feel like opinions are changing and there is some progress, [medicine] still has to deal with the trauma many patients have been through for the past however many years,' she tells me.

'It's one thing for the NICE guidelines to have got rid of treatments like CBT and GET, but I don't feel that's going to end this. We need to deal with the fact a lot of people are terrified, they've been gaslit, they've never been believed,' Jessica adds.

Those living with 'medically unexplained symptoms' who don't yet have a formal diagnosis are at even greater risk of being written off as a hysteric or hypochondriac by the medical establishment. In stark contrast to their progress on the ME treatment guidelines, in 2021 NICE published updated guidelines on the treatment of unexplained chronic pain (known as chronic primary pain). These stated that patients suffering from chronic pain with no known underlying cause should no longer be prescribed painkillers, but should instead be offered exercise, antidepressants, talking therapies and acupuncture. Sound familiar?

The new guidelines were widely condemned by the chronic illness community, not only for their potential to leave patients suffering with unmanaged pain, but for making it even easier for doctors to dismiss 'unexplained' chronic pain as psychological rather than investigating further to find a cause.

*

So, what do we actually now know about women and chronic illness, and where are the gaps that so many of these sick women repeatedly fall through? Underfunding and lack of research are a huge problem for conditions that primarily affect women. ME, chronic migraine, rheumatoid arthritis and MS are all right up there with endometriosis on the list of underfunded, female-dominant conditions. This not only means our understanding of the individual conditions is limited, but there's also a significant gap in our understanding of the links between them and why so many female chronic illness patients develop more than one condition (known as comorbidities) side by side.

Some research is now beginning to delve into these mysteries. Researchers at the University of Oxford, for example, have found genetic correlations between endometriosis and a number of inflammatory autoimmune conditions, including rheumatoid arthritis and osteoarthritis. Recent research published in the *Journal of Clinical Investigation* has suggested that fibromyalgia, which causes chronic widespread pain, may in fact be an autoimmune response, not a condition originating in the brain, as previously believed. Meanwhile, the ongoing DecodeME project is set to be the largest ever biomedical study of ME, seeking to understand whether there's a genetic basis for the disease.

Unlocking the causes of these poorly understood conditions would in turn enable researchers to develop far more effective treatments and diagnostic tools, speeding up diagnosis times and offering patients hope for their quality of life. It could also help to address the question that I personally am so fascinated by: *Why* are women so much more prone to these illnesses than men? So far, though, science can offer little more than theories and speculation.

One theory is that women's more robust immune responses – which make us less likely than men to die from acute infections like Covid-19 – could trigger chronic inflammation and autoimmune diseases. 'Viral infections prompt the immune system to respond. For many women, particularly if they're genetically predisposed, that immune response can be so robust that you enter into this kind of dysregulated immunity, which doesn't get turned off even after the virus is cleared,' Julie Nusbaum, an assistant professor at NYU Long Island School of Medicine, told the *Guardian*.

A number of other theories focus on the role of sex-specific hormones. In autoimmune diseases, for example, researchers DeLisa Fairweather and Noel R. Rose suggest that: 'sex hormones may further amplify this hyperimmune response to infection in susceptible persons, which leads to an increased prevalence of autoimmune diseases in women'. Likewise with ME, fatigue specialist Professor Julia Newton from Newcastle Hospitals tells me: 'My suspicion is that [the gender gap] is, at least in part, related to hormonal changes – but there's no evidence for that yet.'

The same may be true for EDS and hypermobility disorders, multisystem conditions which are typically characterised by 'bendy' joints, stretchy skin, pain and fatigue. 'If you look at symptomatology in children with EDS, [the prevalence by gender] is very similar up until the age of about 10 or 11. But, once puberty kicks in, there's a divergence between males and females, whereby boys tend to improve and girls tend to get worse,' explains Dr Emma Reinhold, a former GP and a researcher specialising in EDS, who lives with the condition herself.

This is believed to be down to the hormonal changes occurring at puberty, with increasing testosterone levels in boys helping to stabilise their connective tissues. For girls, and later women, it's believed to be progesterone which has the most impact, with symptoms worsening premenstrually each month, as well as during pregnancy and menopause.

All these questions come back to the broader issue that science still just doesn't know or understand enough about female hormones. Having historically excluded women and female animals from biomedical research, there are now huge gaps in medicine's understanding of the hormonal mechanisms underlying many female-dominant conditions. Ironically, this exclusion was justified, among other reasons, because our fluctuating hormone cycles were deemed too complicated – an added layer of complexity, and therefore cost, for researchers to account for. Although scientists have since begun to play catch-up, it's maddening to think of the decades of missed opportunities, and all the medical mysteries still yet to be unlocked as a result. Much more truly inclusive research is needed to bridge these gaps and must properly take sex and gender differences into account, including trans status and the effects of hormonal treatments.

From a clinical perspective, the limits of existing research – and the slow rate at which new research findings trickle down to frontline staff – also leave healthcare professionals in a difficult position. While there's never any excuse for dismissing, disbelieving or gaslighting the patient sat in front of you, it's also virtually impossible to diagnose a condition you know nothing about. Even if you can reach an appropriate diagnosis, it's equally challenging to provide effective treatments when very few exist – or, indeed, when the guidelines you've been trained to follow are flawed.

Dr Nina Muirhead, a dermatologist and director of Doctors with ME, has written that she 'didn't believe in' and 'didn't know about or understand' ME prior to being diagnosed with it herself. The NICE guidelines on CBT and GET, she added, had 'perpetuated my misunderstanding of ME/CFS.' After becoming ill, however, she quickly discovered, 'There was no psychological component whatsoever [and] exercise, if anything, was making me worse, not better.'

GP trainee Dr Hannah Barham-Brown was diagnosed with EDS at medical school, after a lecturer noticed her bendy joints and referred her to a colleague in rheumatology. Without that personal experience, though, she suspects she'd be none the wiser about the condition. 'It's not something we're really taught about, because we don't have the research,' she tells me.

As both a doctor and a patient, Hannah says, she's encountered fellow GPs who simply don't believe in her condition. 'Some doctors have very negative attitudes towards EDS. There's still an attitude amongst some that it doesn't really exist, that it's just a diagnosis for people who are slightly bendy and want to pathologise themselves,' she says. 'It's looked upon in the same way that fibromyalgia and ME are, as being this kind of hysterical women's condition.'

While Hannah believes this is primarily down to a simple lack of knowledge and information, she adds: 'There is an ingrained defensiveness in medicine of "me doctor, you patient". I do think we're improving as health professionals and getting better at accepting there are things we don't know, but we really need to keep working to get rid of this attitude. If a patient comes in and says, "I'm specifically worried about this," it's our duty to properly investigate now – even if that means sitting in the uncomfortable space of having to accept your own lack of knowledge, and then going away and learning.'

*

Navigating these difficult dynamics is sadly a fact of life for chronically ill patients. But, as in so many other areas of healthcare, there's also a growing movement of chronic illness advocates and activists, speaking out about their healthcare experiences and fighting for better treatment.

It's worth first pointing out that disability activism, in all its many and varied forms, has a long history as one of the most creative and powerful campaigning movements out there – albeit one that is too frequently overlooked. Over the last few decades, disabled campaigners like Disabled People Against Cuts (DPAC) and the Disabled People's Direct Action Network (DAN) have led radical protests against ableism, inaccessible public services and cuts to health and social care, as well as fighting for better representation.

In 1995, for example, disabled activists staged a string of protests where they handcuffed themselves to buses and trains across the UK to successfully demand more accessible public transport services. More than two decades later, in 2016, the global Millions Missing protest saw a sea of empty shoes arranged outside the UK's Department of Health – and in other locations across the globe – to highlight the millions of ME patients missing from society and call for improvements to research and treatments. Many patients who were too ill to attend in person, like Jessica Taylor-Bearman, sent a pair of their own shoes – a powerful symbol of their absence from the outside world, forced on them by the debilitating nature of their illness.

The internet, though, has undoubtedly galvanised the disability and chronic illness movements, with blogs and social media providing a somewhat more accessible space for sharing information, experiences, rage, companionship and campaigns around the world. Perhaps most significantly it's brought some much-needed intersectionality to a movement that's historically appeared quite homogenous. Social media advocates from a range of backgrounds provide diverse and inclusive perspectives on disability and chronic illness, exploring how issues like racism, homophobia and transphobia, classism, fatphobia, neurodiversity and mental ill health, as well as cultural barriers within different communities, can all intersect with the ableism disabled people face.

Sukhjeen Kaur founded the Chronically Brown community after being diagnosed with rheumatoid arthritis at university, aged just 20. Although Sukhjeen was diagnosed relatively quickly thanks to the severity of her symptoms, she recalls having to cry and plead with doctors before she was taken seriously. 'It started as a pain in my wrist, which they said was just student life – too much writing – and that it would go away. Over the next three months, though, it progressed into my hand, leaving it in a stiff, claw-like shape. I was really struggling, but doctors dismissed me. They said I was too young [for arthritis] and it didn't make any sense; it was just pain. For the first few weeks they genuinely thought I was overreacting and wasting their time,' she says.

After her diagnosis, though, Sukhjeen faced a new challenge in the form of her South Asian extended family. 'South Asians don't talk about disability and chronic illness – there's this attitude that you should be trying harder to get better, or that if they can't see a physical problem then there's nothing actually wrong with you,' she explains. 'My immediate family was very supportive, but certain members of my wider family just started avoiding me. They wouldn't come over to the house or speak to me, and I found the whole situation really, really depressing.'

Sukhjeen initially started her Instagram account in the hope of educating family members about her illness, which she says has helped to some extent, but she soon found that other chronically ill British Asians were getting in touch with their own, similar stories. 'There weren't many white chronic illness spaces actually allowing us to have a voice, so I started sharing these stories on my account and it's really grown from there,' she explains. Chronically Brown has since launched a #Desiabled campaign to destigmatise disability in South Asian communities, as well as running workshops for community elders.

Besides the broader community, Sukhjeen says she's also faced biased assumptions from healthcare staff. 'I'm only 22 and have never mentioned wanting children to my consultant. But she's chosen my medication based on this mentality that, as a young South Asian woman, I'm going to get married and have kids; that's my only worth,' she explains. 'These kinds of attitudes really let us down.'

Hannah Hoskins (@notyourgrandmasuk) is another chronic illness advocate whose activism exists primarily online and is driven, in no small part, by her experiences of navigating the healthcare system. She was diagnosed with fibromyalgia in her mid-20s after being struck down by widespread pain one Christmas. However, despite her GP suggesting fibromyalgia during their first appointment, Hannah initially struggled to get the formal diagnosis she would need to access support. Six years later, in early 2022, Hannah discovered even this was a misdiagnosis, after she was diagnosed instead with subclinical hypothyroidism, an endocrine disorder affecting the production of the thyroid hormone. The hormone treatment she was prescribed for this has, for the first time in years, allowed Hannah to live a relatively pain-free life.

'Before I got sick, I had this idea that [the health and social care system] would be much more organised and structured. Part of my diagnosis was being given a picture of a person and having to colour in where it hurt. That was it!' she says. 'The biggest surprise you face as a newly disabled person is that no one's necessarily going to give you a diagnosis. No one's going to hand you a blue badge and tell you when you've become disabled.'

For Hannah, joining the online disability community gave her the confidence to start customising her mobility aids in her trademark bubblegum pink leopard print designs, having previously felt self-conscious about being visibly disabled in public. It also provided a space for her to speak out about her experiences and in 2019 she began using her background as a TV production manager to create the resources she wished she'd had during those bewildering early days. Today, alongside her educational *No Bull Guide to Chronic Illness*, Hannah also runs her own business, Not Your Grandma's, selling fun, vibrant disability aids and accessories to help people be seen for their personality and not their disability.

Fundamentally though, Hannah hopes that chronic illness newbies can benefit from her experience and research. 'My activism is all about sharing information. I love to research, and I think there's a lot of value in sharing that information and supporting each other,' she explains. 'We can get so fixated on activism in the traditional sense – which isn't always accessible for everyone – but sometimes activism actually starts at home. What I'm doing is providing a platform where people feel stronger to speak out about their experiences, to share and to educate those around them. Of course we need to focus on big structural changes, but it all starts with people just understanding disability better – that, I think, is more important for me.'

Perhaps unsurprisingly, the question of how to deal with doctors is one of the recurring themes in Hannah's conversations with other disabled women. 'Most people think, like I did, that you go to the doctor, tell them what's wrong and they will fix it for you. But sometimes they don't have the answers, sometimes it takes time and a battery of tests for them to understand what's going on,' she explains. 'I also realised that doctors are trained in a very specific way, so understanding the type of language to use and how to approach them can help you to get the best out of that very short window of time you get in your appointments,' she adds.

Hannah's solution was to delve into medical textbooks in search of some insight into what makes healthcare professionals tick. As she wrote in a 2020 guest post for Hysterical Women, 'From the beginning of medical school, doctors are taught about how they themselves might fall foul of the hypochondria narrative – although they call it "medical student syndrome". This, Hannah explained, is a phenomenon where medical students, armed with their newly gained medical knowledge, and under intense pressure to perform, accidentally misdiagnose themselves.

Knowing this, she wrote, 'You can understand that when a patient like us walks into a clinic, having spent time researching what could possibly be the cause of our symptoms, we accidentally set off the red flags. There is an art to getting your doctor to investigate what you think might be happening and it's one so many of us have to learn from scratch.' While this can be exhausting and demoralising in itself, Hannah believes it's at least a little bit easier to navigate with a supportive community behind you. You can find her tips and tricks for getting through healthcare appointments in the toolkit at the end of this chapter.

*

The experiences we've heard about from the disabled and chronically ill women in this chapter are rooted in a deep history of medical misogyny and ignorance, both of which continue to affect women and those assigned female at birth – as well as minority groups – to this day. They also provide some important context for what happened during the Covid-19 pandemic.

From a gendered perspective, throughout the pandemic men have statistically been more likely than women to die from Covid-19. But this fact in isolation only tells part of an incredibly complex story. As in so many other areas of healthcare, the evidence quickly highlighted that people from Black and ethnic minority backgrounds were at disproportionate risk of serious illness or death from Covid-19.

Meanwhile, research highlighted by the Women's Equality Party in 2021 showed disabled women with higher support needs were 91% more likely to die from Covid-19 than the general population. Disabled people more generally had a 'markedly increased' risk of mortality from Covid, making up 60% of Covid deaths to November 2020 despite representing just 17% of the population. The same figures showed that severely disabled people were at more than three times the risk of death and people with learning disabilities as much as eight times more likely to die from the virus.

From the early days in spring 2020, Covid-19 was framed as a disease primarily affecting the elderly and vulnerable – a belief that unleashed all manner of ageism and ableism from lockdown sceptics, not to mention a significant degree of complacency from those who saw themselves as too young and healthy to be affected. I've heard from countless disabled and clinically vulnerable women that attitudes – both from the general public and as part of the wider public health messaging – made them feel 'disposable'.

Perhaps most shocking were reports of disabled patients being pressured by doctors to have Do Not Resuscitate (DNR) orders placed on their medical records or, particularly in the case of people with learning disabilities, being given DNR orders without any prior consultation. A later report commissioned by the Care Quality Commission (CQC) found that 30% of people with a DNR order in place were not aware of it. It's hardly surprising then that disability charity Scope reported 63% of disabled people were concerned they wouldn't get the hospital treatment they needed if they became ill with coronavirus.

Learning disability charity Mencap has been campaigning on this particular health gap since long before the pandemic. In 2007 it published *Death by Indifference,* a report highlighting the avoidable deaths of people with learning disabilities, which was followed up a decade later by its current ongoing Treat Me Well campaign.

According to Mencap, people with learning disabilities have worse physical and mental health, and shorter life expectancies, than people without. This is particularly true for learning-disabled women. The 2018 Learning Disabilities Mortality Review found the median age at death for people with learning disabilities was 60 for men and 59 for women. Compared to the median age of death for people in the general population, this was a difference of 23 years for men and 27 years for women. Pre-Covid, in 2018, Mencap estimated that 1200 learning-disabled people each year died avoidably as a result of healthcare inequalities, including a lack of reasonable adjustments to ensure healthcare is accessible for all.

One of the deaths highlighted in *Death by Indifference* was that of Carole Foster, who died aged 52 in 2006 after her hospital failed to treat her for gallstones. Instead, the report says, 'Staff interpreted the change in her behaviour as symptomatic of her learning disability and mental ill health.' After an ombudsman report in 2011 found that Carole's death had been avoidable, her sister-in-law told the BBC: 'Having learning disabilities, she didn't know what was going on and was a very, very frightened lady. She was being treated like she had broken down with her psychiatric problems, when in fact it was her pain barrier that had broken. She was frightened and hurting, and nobody was listening.'

Ciara Lawrence, who has a learning disability herself and works at Mencap, was a particularly vocal advocate for the care of learning-disabled people throughout the pandemic. 'People with learning disabilities aren't listened to and we're not properly respected, because doctors don't have the right training,' she tells me. 'I've been in appointments where it felt like my voice was taken away and that's not right. Doctors use big, clever words, they rush you and they don't make reasonable adjustments. That doesn't help me. Sadly, we're more likely to die because of these bad attitudes.'

The type of reasonable adjustments Ciara talks about are not complicated: allowing extra time for appointments; using simple, jargon-free language or providing written information in easy-read formats; ensuring the patient has understood everything; and giving them time to ask questions. These are, as Ciara says, 'simple, easy adjustments that can make an awfully big difference' – yet inadequate training and intense time pressures mean too many healthcare professionals are failing to provide the type of care that learning-disabled people really need.

There's no doubt the pandemic has heightened many of the logistical challenges already facing the NHS, but it's also exposed some disturbing attitudes about the value that's placed on disabled lives. In both cases, as always, it's primarily been the most marginalised patients who have paid the price.

*

The other significant and gendered impact of the pandemic has been the emergence of a whole new chronic illness: Long Covid. Much like ME, Long Covid is a post-viral condition, characterised by symptoms that persist for three months or more after the original Covid-19 infection, and it appears to affect more women than men. Also like ME, those affected by it have soon found that their symptoms are dismissed and psychologised as 'stress' or 'anxiety'.

Barbara Melville-Jóhannesson was one of the first Covid 'long haulers' to begin campaigning on the issue in the UK, having caught Covid-19 during the pandemic's first wave. Both she and her partner experienced a 'quite mild' infection in March 2020, before the country had even gone into lockdown. After a couple of weeks, though, he had got better, while Barbara had started to experience breathing difficulties.

As things got worse, with shortness of breath, tightness across the chest and her fingernails turning blue, Barbara made several calls to her GP and NHS 111, as well as presenting at her local out-of-hours centre to be assessed, but to no avail. Her oxygen saturation results were good, which Barbara says felt like 'being gaslighted by the equipment,' and a 111 operator explained that her symptoms weren't 'bad enough' before asking if she suffered from anxiety. It wasn't until Barbara collapsed and an ambulance had to be called that she felt she was really believed and taken seriously.

By late April, Barbara had started to hear and see similar stories to her own, both in hospital and online, and joined a Facebook support group which already had a few hundred members. As more and more people joined, she says, it quickly developed into a movement. 'It was so disorganised because we were all just laying around in our beds, watching the issues that were coming up. I was terrified and clutching at anything that would make me feel a bit safer, but it was amazing to find this group of other sick people, largely women, who were so motivated by our shared vision,' she says. 'We were probably quite naive – none of us had campaigned before and it was very reactive at first, but we had an energy and a fire in our bellies where we just needed to do something.'

Fellow first-wave long hauler Jasmine Hayer was similarly inspired to launch the Hidden Voices of Long Covid, a project curating the stories and experiences of hundreds of Long Covid patients. 'Just as I experienced, countless Long Covid patients are not given the extensive testing they need – their initial tests appear "normal" and their symptoms are written off as "anxiety",' she says. 'But just because there's no evidence for something yet, it doesn't mean it's not there.'

In Jasmine's case, although her initial blood tests and CT scan were clear, subsequent testing revealed a whole range of heart and lung problems, including fluid around her heart, 'post-Covid blood clot phenomena', and abnormal blood flow in her lungs. 'Imagine what could be happening in the bodies of countless patients who are equally being dismissed,' she says. Through her project, by giving a voice to so many people with Long Covid, Jasmine hopes the world will finally listen to the patients at the centre of this hidden and emerging health crisis.

'We're seeing in the clinics that women in their 20s, 30s and 40s are affected most by Long Covid, similar to ME/CFS. I've received over 500 private messages and the majority are from young women who share a very similar story to me – that they were dismissed by their doctor and fobbed off. They used to be very fit and healthy, and many are now so debilitated they cannot work. Hidden Voices echoes this,' she tells me.

By June 2021, more than two million people had been affected by Long Covid since the start of the pandemic, with the type and severity of their symptoms varying wildly. The nature of Covid-19 meant a huge number of people suddenly getting sick, and staying sick, all at once – from a brand-new disease that both researchers and frontline staff were battling to try and understand. Unsurprisingly, with such a keen focus on tackling acute Covid infections, the NHS initially struggled to know what to do with the one in 20 patients who didn't get better again afterwards.

Undoubtedly, though, the historic neglect of ME and other chronic conditions didn't help. Long Covid is a new condition in its own right, with more than 200 symptoms identified across 10 different organ systems, but many of these bear a striking resemblance to existing conditions. Common symptoms include extreme tiredness, post-exertional malaise and cognitive difficulties or 'brain fog', like ME.

Others, like those Barbara experienced, include shortness of breath, heart palpitations, chest pain or tightness and dizziness, all of which are symptoms of PoTS. This is a form of dysautonomia – a disorder of the autonomic nervous system – and is most common in girls and women aged 15–50 or, in other words, those who are menstruating. It's another condition that isn't well-known within the medical profession. According to charity PoTS UK, up to 50% of patients are told their symptoms are 'all in their head' and women with PoTS have told me they regularly have to explain their condition to every new doctor they see.

As a result, therefore, instead of having decades' worth of knowledge, experience and effective treatment pathways to fall back on, the NHS was wholly unprepared for such an influx of long-term sickness and disability. Dr David Strain is a consultant in the Devon ME/CFS service, who has played a leading role in the BMA's response to Long Covid while also living with the condition himself. At a media briefing hosted by charity Action for ME in August 2021, he expressed frustration that the ongoing Long Covid crisis could have been avoided if only the medical community had listened to people with ME a long time ago.

Yet Long Covid could – and frankly must – be a moment of reckoning for the medical community about how all chronic illnesses are prioritised, researched and treated. The large volume of media coverage that Long Covid campaigners have successfully generated, as well as the large number of frontline healthcare professionals affected, mean Long Covid has garnered significantly more public, political and research attention than ME has ever been afforded, including significant NHS investments to set up dedicated Long Covid clinics. As David said, 'There's been more research in the last six months for Long Covid than in the last 10 years for ME.' There's been understandable resentment about this from within the ME community, as well as fear and frustration that history could still end up repeating itself.

Likewise, some women with Long Covid have privately confessed to me that, despite the obvious similarities, they've resisted the ME label in the hope of avoiding the sexism, stigma and psychologisation that's attached to the diagnosis. However, there's already no shortage of reports about Long Covid patients finding themselves disbelieved, told their symptoms are 'all in their head' or advised to try ineffective or harmful treatments like CBT and GET.

Dr Kelly Fearnley, with whom I spoke at a panel event on the psychologisation of physical illnesses, described being treated like 'an anxious little girl' after being taken to A&E with Long Covid symptoms. Despite being a doctor herself, she says there was no help available from her medical colleagues when she needed it – and she's convinced her gender, working-class background, northern accent and junior position as a foundation doctor all played a role in the treatment she received. Meanwhile, Dr Asad Khan, who chaired the panel, said doctors dismissed him as 'stressed', and encouraged him to 'push through' his symptoms with exercise.

As of March 2021, Kelly and Asad were two of more than 100,000 NHS employees affected by Long Covid, with long-term staff sicknesses adding to the already significant pressures on frontline health services. This impact on their medical colleagues, as well as the influx of research interest, provides a golden opportunity for all those within the profession to seriously rethink their attitudes towards chronic illness. 'We could be facing people with ME for decades to come as a result of this pandemic and it's absolutely paramount that we get treatment right; that we don't tell these people it's all in their heads,' says David.

One doctor whose practice has already been shaped by her Long Covid experience is GP Dr Amy Small. She credits people with other chronic illnesses for educating and supporting her through her struggle with Long Covid, and ultimately making her a better doctor. 'Previously when I was faced with a patient who had ME, I would feel hopeless to help them in any which way. I had always been taught they needed CBT and GET to cure this illness, and if they didn't do that they weren't really trying hard enough,' she explains.

'I've had consultations recently that were totally different from how I would have done them before getting sick and learning from the chronic illness community, so I'm definitely a better doctor for it. There's so much I didn't really understand and so much we can all learn from each other,' Amy adds. 'What I'm doing now is lobbying for better care for people with Long Covid. If we can get this right for Long Covid then we can get it right for all chronic illnesses. Everyone with ME, fibromyalgia, rheumatoid arthritis, MS and so on needs proper support from a multidisciplinary team.'

YOUR CHRONIC ILLNESS AND DISABILITY TOOLKIT

Alas, I don't have any easy solutions for the big and complex problems we've addressed in this chapter. If you're reading this with a large stash of cash that you're not sure what to do with, an investment in redressing some of these gaping research gaps certainly wouldn't go amiss.

In the meantime, Hannah Hoskins has kindly shared her advice for navigating the healthcare system when you're disabled or chronically ill. 'A lot of it is understanding the best way to speak to doctors and the kind of language to use,' she says. Doctors are taught to consider a patient's ideas, concerns and expectations (the ICE model), and this is a useful framework to keep in mind when preparing for your appointments. 'I always suggest taking emotional language out of the conversation and being very practical in the way you talk about it – "this bit hurts and it causes me this issue". It's difficult because these conditions can be a very emotional experience, but unfortunately you only get 5–10 minutes and if there's any emotion it just gives the doctor a tool to discount you,' Hannah adds.

This, she says, is undoubtedly a gendered issue and, sad as it is, another of her top tips is always to 'take a bloke' to your appointments if possible. 'I experimented and found I was actually listened to a lot more when my partner was present. He didn't even have to say anything, he was often just sat staring at his shoes, but there was a complete change in the dynamic.'

Even if you don't have a suitable man to accompany you, Hannah says two people are always better than one – go with a relative, friend, carer or whoever has your back. 'Having two people is really helpful because the other person can confirm what was said and act almost like a witness,' she explains. 'It's a gentle way of asserting yourself and making it clear that you're there to be taken seriously. Unfortunately, it's all a game of power play, language and personalities, and it can be quite difficult to balance them all.'

When it comes to feeling empowered about taking control of your own health, Hannah's a big advocate of getting a copy of your medical records and being proactive about keeping track of everything that's said at each appointment. 'It's also worth asking your doctor whether they've dealt with chronically ill patients before and don't be afraid to request someone different if they turn out to be shit,' she says.

Of course, all of this requires huge amounts of resilience and persistence, with little guarantee that you'll get the answers or treatments you need. This is tough, but it's absolutely no reflection on you. 'There are periods where I don't fight because it's easier and you can't beat yourself up in those periods either,' Hannah says. 'Sometimes you do just get too sick and don't have the energy; you have to find a balance. The main thing is finding a community that will support you in whatever way you need to be supported, where you can feel comfortable enough to talk openly about your own experience. Any activism and advocacy can follow on from that.'

Resources
- Action for ME – actionforme.org.uk
- Arthritis Action – arthritisaction.org.uk
- British Pain Society – britishpainsociety.org
- Chronically Awesome – chronicallyawesome.org.uk
- Chronically Brown – chronicallybrown.com
- Ehlers-Danlos Support UK – ehlers-danlos.org
- Fibromyalgia Action UK – fmauk.org
- Guts UK – gutscharity.org.uk
- Long Covid Support – longcovid.org
- Lupus UK – lupusuk.org.uk
- Mast Cell Action – mastcellaction.org
- ME Association – meassociation.org.uk
- ME Trust – metrust.org.uk
- Mencap – mencap.org.uk
- MS Society – mssociety.org.uk
- Multiple Sclerosis Trust – mstrust.org.uk
- Not Your Grandma's – notyourgrandmas.co.uk
- PoTS UK – potsuk.org
- Scope – scope.org.uk
- Versus Arthritis – versusarthritis.org

5

'All in your head': Mental health and hysteria

Content note: This chapter discusses trauma, self-harm and suicide. If these topics are triggering for you, please skip ahead.

Women's mental health is a thorny issue in feminist criticism. There's no doubt that sexism and other biases are as pervasive in psychiatric diagnosis as they are elsewhere in medicine. We know, for example, about psychiatry's history of branding difficult women 'mad' or 'hysterical'. During the Victorian era, such women were shoved out of the way in asylums or locked in attics, simply for failing to conform to society's expectations of them – for transgressions like showing an 'excess of emotion' or, god forbid, disobeying their husbands.

Over the last couple of centuries, women's emotions and their ways of expressing them have been viewed both as inherently problematic and as evidence of their natural 'irrationality' compared to men. Meanwhile, feminist critics like Elaine Showalter, author of *The Female Malady*, and psychotherapists like Phyllis Chesler have reframed historic descriptions of women's 'madness' as both an expression of and a rebellion against female powerlessness.

In the 2005 edition of her 1972 book *Women and Madness*, Phyllis Chesler writes: 'In my time, we were taught to view women as somehow naturally mentally ill. Women were hysterics, malingerers, child-like, manipulative, either cold or smothering as mothers, and driven to excess by their hormones... Although there has been enormous progress, the clinical biases that I first wrote about in 1972 still exist today. Many clinical judgements remain clouded by classism, racism, anti-Semitism, homophobia, ageism, sexism, and by cultural and anti-immigration biases as well.'

Indeed, as Drs Paula J Caplan and Lisa Cosgrove point out in their 2004 book *Bias in Psychiatric Diagnosis,* official diagnostic criteria have long been decided upon by a 'small number of primarily white, high-status, male psychiatrists who... have had more power than any group to decide who is and is not psychologically normal.' As a result, it's possible that disparities in psychiatric diagnoses may, at least in part, come down to over-diagnosis and an ongoing tendency to pathologise difference.

Women are more likely than men to be diagnosed with common mental health issues like depression and anxiety, as well as eating disorders and PTSD, despite the latter's persistent association with (mostly male) war veterans. The controversial diagnosis of borderline or emotionally unstable personality disorder (BPD/EUPD) is overwhelmingly applied to women, while Black patients are disproportionately diagnosed with stigmatised conditions like schizophrenia.

Psychiatric medication like antidepressants and anti-anxiety drugs are also more likely to be prescribed to women, with sedative diazepam (Valium) colloquially referred to as 'mother's little helper'. Meanwhile, men are believed to be more likely than women to under-report their struggles with mental ill health, putting off seeking help and instead self-medicating using recreational drugs and alcohol, or expressing their emotions in more physical ways like violence and aggression.

Even taking over-diagnosis into account, though, both research and anecdotal evidence make it clear that women and minority groups *are* disproportionately affected by emotional distress. According to NHS data, mental ill health among women is on the rise, with one in five (19%) affected by a common mental health issue like depression or anxiety, compared to one in eight men. Young women (aged 16–24) are the group at highest risk of mental ill health and a quarter (26%) of women in this age group have self-harmed – more than twice the number of young men.

For those affected by multiple disadvantages, rates of mental ill health are higher still with 29% of Black women, 24% of Asian women and 29% of mixed-race women affected by common mental health problems. Among LGBTQ+ communities, research by Stonewall shows staggeringly high rates of depression and anxiety, particularly among lesbian and bisexual women, trans and non-binary people: 55% of lesbian and bisexual women experience depression and 65% anxiety, while around 70% of trans and non-binary people experience one or both.

Unsurprisingly, bias, minority stress and socioeconomic factors play a significant role in these rates of mental ill health. Women who experience sexism are more likely to develop mental health issues, while additional experiences of discrimination like racism, homophobia, transphobia and ableism have similar exacerbating effects. Within these conversations, it's therefore important to bear in mind that the mental health challenges faced by a white, cis, heterosexual, comfortably well-off, middle-class woman may well look very different from those faced by a queer, Black, working-class trans woman without access to stable housing or employment.

As Daniel and Jason Freeman, authors of *The Stressed Sex*, note: 'Social stresses make people vulnerable to mental illness and research indicates that women's roles may be especially demanding. Considering that on the whole women are paid less, find it harder to advance in a career, have to juggle multiple roles, and are bombarded with images of apparent female "perfection", it would be amazing if there wasn't some emotional cost.' Women are also twice as likely as men to have experienced trauma from interpersonal violence and abuse. Research by charity Agenda shows that more than 50% of women who've experienced 'extensive physical and sexual violence' have a common mental health condition, while one in three have attempted suicide.

Ironically, though, given the historic tendency to pathologise and medicalise women's emotional states, they also struggle to be taken seriously and access appropriate care; dismissed, instead, as 'drama queens' and 'attention seekers' or told that 'all women are emotional'. There are obvious links between the normalisation of women's physical pain – as with endometriosis, for example – and this normalisation of their psychological distress, even at crisis point.

Molly tells me about seeking help from her GP for low mood, self-harm, suicidal thoughts and severe anxiety from the age of just 14. 'Throughout my teenage years I was told by various GPs that "All teenage girls struggle with their mood." This was in spite of them knowing I was experiencing abuse, but they never considered it might be related,' she says. Similarly, Hysterical Women contributor Rachel recalls her self-harm being dismissed as 'a teenage phase'. When she subsequently attempted suicide at 18, she adds, 'No one queried it further. I think everyone thought I was just doing these things for attention. Some went so far as to tell me that directly, but I am sure many more were thinking it.'

Much has been said, particularly in recent years, about the urgent need to tackle the alarming male suicide rate. Suicide is the biggest killer of men under 45 and there is no doubt that this is a crisis – and a gendered one at that. Toxic masculinity and a fear of asking for help or being perceived as weak can be significant barriers to men accessing mental healthcare before it's too late. Campaigns like CALM (the Campaign Against Living Miserably) have been influential in highlighting these issues, and the mental health sector is understandably now more mindful of ensuring that men who do reach out are taken seriously and supported at the first available opportunity.

But it's also important to consider the so-called 'suicide gender paradox', which paints a more complex picture. Research consistently shows that, although men are more likely to die from their attempts, women actually attempt suicide at higher rates. At least part of the reason for the paradox is that men typically use more violent methods of suicide, meaning they are more likely to complete their suicide before anyone can intervene. Consequently, though, while male suicide is rightly treated as a tragedy, women's suicidal thoughts, feelings and behaviours are too often written off as not being a credible enough risk to take them seriously.

There's something particularly pernicious about the type of language that is used in these cases – phrases like 'attention-seeking' and 'cry for help' – as if a 'failed' or non-fatal suicide attempt is not a good enough reason to sit up and pay attention or indeed to provide the support that patient desperately needs. Not only that, but data from the Office for National Statistics (ONS) showed that, in 2019, the suicide rate for women and girls was at its highest since 2004. Those aged 50–54 were most at risk, but the data also showed a sharp rise in suicides among girls and young women aged 10–24, up 94% since 2012. Do women have to start dying at the same rates as men before these 'cries for help' are taken seriously?

*

There is, of course, a broader issue of lack of resourcing. Chronic underfunding of NHS mental health services means waiting lists for support are months or, in some areas, even years long. Research published by the Royal College of Psychiatrists in 2020 found that patients with severe mental illnesses – including eating disorders, bipolar disorder and PTSD – were left waiting up to two years for treatment, while others waited up to four years for treatment for depression, anxiety and suicidal thoughts.

Two-fifths of patients were forced to contact emergency or crisis services in the meantime, while more than 10% ended up in A&E. Anecdotally, I've heard from women – including mothers of mentally unwell children and teenagers – who had been told referrals to mental health services wouldn't even be accepted unless there had already been a suicide attempt.

Clearly there's a very dangerous false economy in making people wait until they've reached crisis point before, if they're lucky, help becomes available. Faced with these waiting lists, though, many GPs may understandably feel their hands are tied – that beyond prescribing antidepressants and handing out helpline numbers there's nothing more they can do. These resourcing challenges affect all patients to some extent, but, as is so often the case, women and other marginalised groups face additional barriers and biases within the system.

It's not just sexist stereotypes about 'emotional' and 'hysterical' women that persist. Just as racist myths about 'thicker skin' and 'higher pain thresholds' result in Black women's physical pain being dismissed, stereotypes like the 'strong Black woman' can be a further barrier to mental health support. Indeed, racism within the healthcare system itself means that while Black British adults experience the most severe mental health symptoms, they're the least likely to receive treatment – yet are four times more likely to be detained (sectioned) under the Mental Health Act.

There's also a serious problem about the suitability of care that's on offer and the training therapists receive (or rather, don't receive) to equip them for working sensitively with marginalised patients. 'Within the NHS system, for some reason, Black people are notoriously believed to be stronger and therefore are more likely to have their health concerns dismissed,' explains Soraya Stuart, speaking at the time as a host for Black Minds Matter UK – an organisation set up in the wake of George Floyd's murder in 2020 to provide free therapy, with Black therapists, to Black individuals and families.

'When it comes to the therapy needs of Black people, generally the NHS only really caters to mild to moderate traumas. It's not really directed towards Black people who suffer more from complex PTSD, as well as inherited and secondary traumas. CBT isn't necessarily going to help us overcome things like systemic racism,' she adds. Equally, Soraya explains, Black Minds Matter's decision only to work with Black therapists was based on the lack of cultural sensitivity and understanding – as well as both implicit and explicit racial bias – that Black patients often encounter from white therapists within the mental health sector.

Unsurprisingly, there has been huge demand for Black Minds Matter's services. After raising half a million pounds in a matter of months they were able to fund therapy for 1200 people, but when Soraya and I spoke in October 2020 there were still 2600 people on their waiting list. While organisations like Black Minds Matter are doing an incredible job, it shouldn't be up to charity and crowdfunding campaigns to pick up the pieces of Black British mental health – and yet the reality in too many areas is an NHS system that's struggling even to cope with the basics.

For trans and non-binary patients, too, the phenomenon of trans broken arm syndrome that we explored earlier is just as applicable to mental healthcare, if not more so. 'Many mental health service providers appear to regard trans people's mental health as relevant only in terms of or in relation to transition,' writes Dr Ruth Pearce, author of *Understanding Trans Health*. 'This means that support for mental health issues unrelated to transition may be difficult for patients to access.'

Even when they are able to access support, she adds, trans patients may find their trans identity raised unnecessarily. Michelle tells me about seeking therapy following a suicide attempt, only to face questioning about her body that was irrelevant, but also horrifyingly intrusive and inappropriate. 'I was there to talk about my mental health, including trauma from my childhood, but the psychologist cut in and asked how I felt about my genitals. I said I didn't want to talk about that, because it wasn't relevant to why I was there, but she tried to make the whole session about my genitals. Presumably she thought it was related because I'm trans,' she says.

'What we really need is for all NHS therapists to receive regular, mandatory training on providing care that is queer-affirming and trans-affirming, as well as actively anti-racist,' says Sam (not their real name), a queer, non-binary femme who has struggled to access appropriate support for their mental health for years. 'I've often felt like I had to leave the queer part of myself outside of the therapy room. That obviously isn't possible because it's part of me and is intertwined with so many different aspects of my mental health and experiences,' they explain. 'When my queer identity has come up, though, I've either felt dismissed or invalidated, or else I've had to educate straight, cisgender counsellors about queer issues, which feels like such a burden when I'm supposed to be there for support.'

Having previously worked in child and adolescent mental health services (CAMHS), Sam has witnessed this lack of training and awareness, as well as more explicit biases, in their own colleagues. 'I'm not a therapist, but if there was a child who they thought might be exploring their gender or sexuality, I'd always be the person who therapists came to [to] ask about it. I also later found out one of the therapists was openly transphobic on Twitter. This was someone who'd been employed by the NHS to work with children, some of whom could be trans or gender-nonconforming,' they say.

In this day and age, Sam adds, the NHS should be ensuring its therapists don't hold explicit biases against any of their potential patients and that they're actively working to be anti-discriminatory. 'This should be incorporated as standard into their training, just like the mandatory safeguarding training that has to be done every year.'

But, while improving training and education for existing therapists is one thing, there's also a serious issue around access to the profession for those from more diverse backgrounds. 'I'd love to become a therapist myself, but, coming from a working-class background, I'm having to go down the children's nursing route because I just can't afford to train as a therapist. The cost and then lack of support throughout the training process can be huge barriers to working-class people, people of colour, queer and trans people to go into therapy,' Sam explains.

'It seems to largely be a white middle-class playground and anyone else is on the margins. In an ideal world, people from marginalised backgrounds would be able to choose a therapist from a similar background, who has first-hand life experience of the issues they're talking about,' they add.

This is also an issue higher up the chain of command. Mushtag Kahin is a registered nursing associate and mental health practitioner for an NHS Addictions Recovery Community, and she believes a huge part of the problem stems from the lack of diversity in management roles. 'There is a lot of nepotism and discrimination in senior leadership, which impacts patient care, accessibility and who makes the decisions. If the people on the boards don't have insight, empathy or knowledge of marginalised communities and their needs, they can't make mental health services more inclusive,' she says.

'I always say there are no "hard to reach" communities, only hard to reach services,' Mushtag adds. 'If staff at any level of mental healthcare lack empathy and cultural competence, that makes people fearful, so they are less likely to access mental health services. Ethnic minorities especially tend to only come into services at crisis point or under section, because there isn't enough preventative work being done. That's generally not a good experience that will encourage them to seek help again.'

*

As I mentioned earlier, the diagnosis of borderline personality disorder (now also known as emotionally unstable personality disorder) is one of the most striking examples of the ways in which women's emotions continue to be pathologised and attributed to personality flaws, rather than being treated as normal, understandable responses to trauma.

It's for this reason that BPD/EUPD is a controversial diagnosis. Women make up 75% of those diagnosed with BPD, and childhood traumas like abuse and neglect have been identified as particular risk factors. But, while some women find the BPD label useful for giving a name and treatment plan to their experiences, others feel it's unhelpful to have their difficulties put down to a 'disordered' personality. For Phoebe (not her real name), at least at first, the diagnosis was a bit of both.

'I didn't mind the BPD diagnosis so much. I'd spent years being diagnosed with anxiety or depression and I'd pushed the GP [for a more appropriate diagnosis], because I knew something else was going on; it wasn't just anxiety,' she says. 'What changed was I became a feminist and was able to unpack how I was treated.'

Phoebe had been physically and verbally abused throughout her childhood. 'By the time I was about 12 I already had signs of severe depression and an eating disorder, and it escalated from there. I went to the doctor when I was 14 and explained my history; that I'd been beaten up by an alcoholic parent every single day of my life. She looked at me for about 20 seconds, then did this kind of sweeping, dismissive gesture with her arm and told me to look in the paper for therapists. How did she think a teenager was going to pay for that?' she recalls.

This was the beginning of what Phoebe describes as 'decades of gaslighting from GPs' until, in her mid-30s, she experienced a severe mental breakdown and psychotic episode. It was only after this that Phoebe eventually found a GP who took her seriously. 'In the past I'd been told I was lying and making it up, or asked if it was my periods. But that breakdown was really the straw that broke the camel's back and I insisted on seeing several different doctors until someone really listened,' she explains. 'By then I was older, I probably presented a bit less working class than in the past and, even though I was in a really bad situation, my ability to speak and advocate for myself had changed. It was only because I pushed my GP that I did eventually get that diagnosis.'

In that sense, finally being diagnosed with BPD came as something of a relief – a recognition that Phoebe's struggles were real and valid, and a way of naming and potentially treating those issues. In reality, though, when Phoebe was eventually referred to a treatment programme two years later, she found it 'very sexist, deeply problematic and a bit of a cult'.

'It was very much geared around the concept of you being over-emotional, too loud, too overtly angry. There was no recognition that your anger might be justified or any attempt to deal with the cause of that anger. As a woman, you were "cured" if you were controlled into behaving in a way that was less emotional, less loud, less angry – more how women "should" behave,' Phoebe explains.

'It was gaslighting really and it reinforced a lot of the abusive tropes that people growing up with abusive parents are already very used to: being told our feelings weren't valid; that it was our fault; our behaviour was to blame; that we should behave in a certain way instead,' she adds. 'I really think it's the diagnosis that most harks back to the times when they would have just stuck us in asylums for being women who weren't behaving in the way that we should.'

One school of thought is that many of those currently diagnosed with BPD should actually be diagnosed with complex PTSD – a form of PTSD caused by sustained experiences of extreme trauma, abuse and neglect, rather than single traumatic incidents. Academic debates on this issue have raged for decades with complex PTSD only recently beginning to be recognised as a condition in its own right.

As one 2019 *Guardian* article explained: 'BPD and complex PTSD are different disorders, but have similar symptoms. But one major indicator sets them apart: the latest research shows that BPD is 55% inherited whereas complex PTSD is not caused by genetics, but prolonged exposure to traumatic events, usually in childhood… This misdiagnosis affects [abuse] survivors more than anyone else, because they commonly display the psychiatric symptoms common to both disorders, such as anxiety, mood swings, depression, emptiness and displaced anger.'

The reason this can be so harmful is that being labelled with BPD suggests the problem is within the survivor's personality, rather than a result of their traumatic experiences, as clinical psychologist Gillian Proctor explains in the same article. Meanwhile, others interviewed by the *Guardian* highlight the broader sexism associated with the diagnosis. Glyn Lewis, head of psychiatry at University College London, says BPD has become associated with a 'parody of supposed feminine characteristics' and psychotherapist Sly Sarkisova describes it as 'a label that is often misused and applied especially to women, or people who were assigned female at birth, to pathologise them for emotional expressions of suffering.'

When it comes to treatment, too, occupational therapist Keir Harding tells me: 'People who get the diagnosis of BPD, similar to people who might be addicted to alcohol or have an eating disorder, are treated with this attitude of "Well, just stop doing what you're doing." [As mental health professionals] we're used to people who we can step in with, be very paternalistic and controlling towards, and help them get back to some kind of normality. But with this population of people, we're not sure what to do.'

This, he says, can become particularly toxic when patients expressing difficult emotions are dismissed as 'inappropriate' and their past experiences are ignored. 'This happens with women all the time. People diagnosed with BPD have generally been hurt by other people in the past, but often those feelings of anger are pathologised and we will force people to stop doing things,' Keir explains.

'If someone's anger is directed at themselves, you force them to stop hurting themselves – so you'll get three people holding down a sexual assault survivor, removing their clothes and injecting them, and they'll keep doing that until that patient "recovers". If you actually stop and think about that, this cannot be a good way to respond to people who have been assaulted in the past. The power dynamic is so skewed.'

Equally, he adds, the sexist stereotypes that surround the BPD label – terms like 'drama queen', 'manipulative' and 'attention-seeking' – put patients at a disadvantage from the off. 'If you walk into a place that's supposed to help you and the people behind the counter already see you as attention-seeking or manipulative, it's going to take away the legitimacy of anything you're saying or asking for,' he says. This kind of testimonial injustice results in mental health professionals not really listening to what their patients are saying, Keir explains, because everything is seen as stemming from their personality disorder rather than their legitimate experiences.

*

It's also been suggested that BPD may be a misdiagnosis that's applied to neurodiverse women – that is, those with cognitive differences like autism or ADHD (attention deficit hyperactivity disorder). Recent studies have found overlaps between traits associated with autism and ADHD and those associated with BPD, suggesting the conditions could either coexist or be mistaken for each other in some patients.

The first of these papers, conducted by researchers at Cambridge University, looked at overlapping behaviour traits of people diagnosed with BPD and autism. Its lead researcher, Dr Robert Dudas, had met patients with BPD who believed they had been misdiagnosed including, increasingly, patients who believed they were really autistic. 'I think in a number of cases, that is true. They may have been misdiagnosed,' he said. 'Patients have been saying this for a long time and it's really important to do some more detailed studies to look into this.'

Notably, while BPD may be over-diagnosed in women, both autism and ADHD are significantly under-diagnosed in women and girls, largely thanks to gendered stereotypes about who they affect and how. Studies on the gender ratio of autistic males to females, for example, suggest rates ranging from 2:1 to 16:1, with 3:1 currently considered the most up-to-date estimate. Although an increasing amount of attention has been paid to neurodiversity among women in recent years, conditions like autistic spectrum disorders (ASD) and ADHD remain primarily viewed as 'male' conditions, commonly associated, respectively, with socially awkward but gifted men and disruptive, hyperactive schoolboys.

Besides this persistent gender stereotyping, research suggests part of the difficulty with diagnosis is that autistic women and women with ADHD present differently from their male counterparts and are more adept at 'masking' or learning more 'socially acceptable' behaviours. This can equally take its toll on their mental health and self-esteem, leading to secondary issues like depression, anxiety and self-harm.

A 2012 survey by the National Autistic Society found that 42% of women and girls had been diagnosed with psychiatric, personality or eating disorders prior to receiving their autism diagnosis, compared to 30% of men and boys. Similarly with ADHD, girls are more likely to demonstrate 'inattentiveness' than the other ADHD traits of hyperactivity or impulsivity and to be misdiagnosed (or only diagnosed) with mental health issues like anxiety, depression or bipolar disorder.

Author Rebecca Schiller, who is better known for her work on pregnancy and birth, writes movingly about her mental breakdown and the ADHD diagnosis it led to in her memoir *Earthed*. In an interview with Hysterical Women, she tells me: 'When women are hyperactive, the movements they make are very small and socially acceptable, quite feminised – it's a hair twiddle, a skirt rustle. I have learned since I was tiny to be very good at hiding it.' For her, though, getting an appropriate diagnosis has made a huge difference to understanding and processing why she has struggled emotionally with the 'imperative for me to be a functioning, well-behaved, organised, capable person.'

Similarly, retired assistant headteacher Jane Green, who was only diagnosed as autistic at the age of 54, believes gender stereotyping, male spectrum bias and her professional status prevented her from being diagnosed earlier. 'I knew I was different, but I wasn't believed,' she says. 'I was not masking, but I was told, "You can't be autistic, because you're professional, you look normal and you don't love data." I didn't fit into the autistic world, I didn't display what many believe to be the characteristics of an autistic person, but I wanted closure.'

Rebecca describes this struggle to be heard as like being repeatedly rubbed out. 'Mental health is such a fundamental thing about your existence,' she adds. 'There's a trauma in not being listened to that goes beyond just, "I need this treatment and I'm not getting it."' Much more needs to be done to tackle this gender bias, ensuring neurodiverse women and girls are diagnosed, and can access treatment as appropriate, at the earliest possible opportunity. But it's also clear, yet again, that the pressure to conform to gendered expectations can and does have a significant impact on the mental health of any woman who fails to fit neatly into the mould.

*

Eating disorders are another highly gendered and stigmatised area of mental health. Despite as many as a quarter of those affected being men, the stereotypical image of a (usually white, invariably emaciated) young woman persists in our cultural imagination. The full picture is that an estimated 1.25 million people in the UK have an eating disorder, including people of all races, genders, sexualities, socioeconomic backgrounds and, indeed, body shapes and sizes.

Despite this, 2019 research commissioned by eating disorder charity Beat found that the prevailing stereotype prevents people from Black, ethnic minority, and LGBTQ+ communities, as well as people from less affluent backgrounds, from seeking and receiving medical treatment. NHS data from 2017 to 2020 shows a 216% increase in hospital admissions for eating disorders among Black patients, compared to an overall 53% increase for all Black and ethnic minority patients and a 31% increase for white patients. Meanwhile, though, Black people and people of colour felt less confident than white people about seeking medical help for an eating disorder. Just 52% of Black and ethnic minority respondents said they would feel confident doing so, compared to 64% of white British respondents. As the staggering increase in hospital admissions for Black patients shows, much more must urgently be done to provide earlier interventions. Similarly, despite LGBTQ+ people having an increased risk of eating disorders, 37% of LGBTQ+ respondents said they would not feel confident seeking help, compared to just 24% of heterosexual respondents.

Even for women who are able to access medical support for their eating disorders, sexist stereotypes and stigmas are often deeply embedded within these services. Sarah developed severe anorexia in her teens, which she now believes was a coping mechanism for the pain of her undiagnosed and untreated endometriosis. 'Any time I went to the doctor about my endometriosis symptoms they were brushed off – nobody cared. I didn't find out I had endometriosis until years later, but I developed anorexia as a distraction method to manage my symptoms,' she says. 'I was at an all-girls school in Belfast in the early noughties, during the size zero era, and so not eating was very normalised in teenage girls – including by my teachers, who saw it as a running joke that I never ate lunch.'

When Sarah's illness got so severe that she was hospitalised, she experienced what she describes as her first encounter with sexism in medicine – something she'd later become very familiar with. 'My mother was instantly singled out as the cause of my eating disorder. The nurses would very openly make comments, saying I had anorexia because my mum wouldn't let me grow up, or that she was overbearing and controlling because she would make meals for me to eat and bring them in. Actually, my mum was the one who helped me to start eating again,' she says.

Later, in therapy, Sarah came up against another mother-blaming theory – that her anorexia was caused by her mum's failure to correctly perform femininity. 'Mum was a feminist who didn't wear makeup or feminine clothes. She was the breadwinner at home and didn't do any of the household chores.

My therapist had this idea that maybe I was anorexic because I didn't know how to be a woman, because my mother had never shown me how to be one,' Sarah explains. 'I stopped going to therapy after that, because I was so clear that wasn't the cause and this wasn't helping me.'

It's also worth noting that weight stigma in eating disorder services often leaves patients in larger bodies struggling to be taken seriously or even pushes them towards restrictive diets that fuel their disordered eating. According to Beat, anorexia accounts for just 8% of all eating disorder diagnoses in the UK, while binge eating disorder is the most common, making up 22% of cases.

Meg, who I interviewed in 2019, began struggling with binge eating disorder at the age of 17, after a lifetime of pressure to lose weight from parents who restricted her diet. Despite this, it took her 10 years to access treatment for her eating disorder, because so much emphasis was placed on her size rather than her mental health.

'It was very motivated by weight. A lot of people who have binge eating disorder don't necessarily recognise it and doctors don't necessarily probe for it,' she explained. 'When I was 28, I had to be really insistent with my doctor and say, "Look, I've tried this, I've tried that." I feel like you have to pay your dues with lots of failed diets first and then you can say, "Look, I've tried fixing my body, now I have to try to fix my mind, because that's obviously the problem."'

Likewise, patients with anorexia, bulimia and other eating disorders face a battle for timely and appropriate treatment, which is still too often restricted by the health service's unhealthy obsession with BMI and physical appearances. Although NICE guidelines state that BMI should never be the sole measure of the severity of someone's eating disorder, campaigner Hope Virgo was refused treatment for an anorexia relapse on the basis that her BMI was 'healthy' – despite the fact she knew her behaviour was anything but.

Writing for Hysterical Women, Hope described leaving that appointment wondering: 'So what am I? A fake anorexic? A drama queen? An attention-seeker? How can I show you I am really struggling?' As a result of her experience Hope launched the #DumpTheScales campaign, with a petition – which now has more than 100,000 signatures – calling on NHS mental health services to stop relying on weight and BMI, and instead ensure anyone with an eating disorder can access the support they need.

These restrictions on services undoubtedly affect all patients to some extent, but they are not entirely gender-neutral either. As Dr Asher Larmie explained in chapter 3, women are disproportionately affected by weight stigma and judgements on their physical appearances – and this applies at both ends of the BMI scale. 'Eating disorders are not physical illnesses, but they are one of the few mental illnesses where so much is judged on physical appearance and physique,' Hope writes. These judgements are not just unhelpful and unscientific, they're also dangerous – particularly when they encourage disordered eating and unhealthy weight loss for the sole purpose of becoming 'thin enough' to access treatment.

*

The complexities of the relationship between mental and physical health are, as Hope describes, too often simplistically understood by healthcare professionals. This seems to stem from a tendency to see the two as distinct and unconnected – to view eating disorders purely in terms of physical weight, for example, or to overlook the fact that many other mental health conditions, like depression and anxiety, have very real physical effects as well.

In the previous chapter I described the reluctance among many disabled and chronically ill women to seek help for their mental health struggles, largely out of a fear that this would lead to their physical symptoms being dismissed as psychological. Sadly, stories I've heard from women on the other side of the fence suggest this fear may well be justified.

Writing for Hysterical Women, Ruth describes feeling judged as a 'middle-aged mental health patient' after developing very physical symptoms. 'I knew I had fibromyalgia when I went to see my then-GP, because of all the symptoms I was experiencing: pain in every muscle, ligament and tendon from head to toe; burning in my muscles; strange electric shocks; fatigue; poor sleep; brain fog; and a host of other symptoms. But I was met with prejudgment and bias as a woman with a long mental health history,' she writes.

Having researched fibromyalgia and typed up a list of her symptoms, Ruth was astonished by the dismissive reaction from her GP, who simply told her: 'It's surprising what the mind can make the body think it's got.' Years later she sought out a second opinion and, despite her GP's reference to 'psychosomatic symptoms' in the referral letter, a rheumatologist confirmed the diagnosis of fibromyalgia. 'I was disgusted with my GP frankly,' Ruth says. 'He'd just looked at me and gone: "Middle-aged woman, mental health patient, invented syndrome" and dismissed me.'

My friend Philippa describes a similar experience after she woke up one morning with tingling in one leg. Within a few weeks she had tingling and pain in both legs and was referred to a neurologist, who found evidence of unexplained nerve damage – yet her GP's response was: 'At least now we know you're not making it up.' Up until that moment, she hadn't known he disbelieved her. 'I froze. I knew exactly what he was getting at,' she says. 'The long list of psychiatric drugs on my meds list and a long history of various manifestations of madness meant he'd thought I had invented some weird symptoms. Why? Who knows? But he had believed that was the case until the needles stuck into my muscles proved otherwise.'

We know that mental and physical health are interconnected, with each influencing the other in a variety of ways, not least because living with any kind of long-term ill health inevitably has a more widespread impact on both your physical and psychological wellbeing. However, as we've seen, this mistrust of women's ability to understand and accurately report their own symptoms too often forces us to think and talk about them in more binary terms. 'The distinction between body and brain is one we've made up. We've created this very false dichotomy in medicine, and we've done ourselves and our patients a great disservice by allowing [mental and physical health] to be separated,' says disabled GP trainee Dr Hannah Barham-Brown.

'We need both to be working in conjunction and, if they're not, that's when you're going to experience pain or mental health issues and that's going to be difficult to live with,' she explains. 'I often say to patients, "Have you had some mental health support?" Because even if your symptoms are not caused by your mental health issues, and even if you don't think you have any mental health issues, it's going to be hard mentally. Breaking down the body/brain barrier is something we're really bad at.'

This, too, is something Sarah has discovered. Having recovered from anorexia, she has since been diagnosed with three chronic illnesses: endometriosis, adenomyosis and Crohn's disease, a form of inflammatory bowel disease (IBD). 'I'm still struggling to access mental health support, which is just atrocious in Northern Ireland. I've been on a waiting list for psychological services for 18 months, and I've recently been told it'll be another three years for my first appointment,' she tells me.

'I've also been told I'm not allowed to talk about any of my [physical] health issues as part of my psychology appointments. So I can talk about anxiety, I can talk about depression, but I cannot talk about my illnesses and how they affect me because that's a different department,' Sarah explains. 'If I want to talk about pain psychology, I need a separate referral from a pain consultant. I've already been on a waiting list to see them since 2018, so right now I'm stuck. There's no connection, no joined-up thinking, and that really does impact on women, because we're the ones who are primarily dealing with the psychological effects of chronic pain.'

YOUR MENTAL HEALTH TOOLKIT

Again, the chronic underfunding and under-resourcing of mental health services make this a really tricky one. I won't pretend there are easy answers, quick fixes or that anything you can do will magically get you better care.

It's worth checking the list of GPs on your surgery's website to see if any of them have a particular interest or training in mental health, as this may help to ensure you get the most supportive and helpful reception. Failing that, remember that you can always ask to see another doctor for a second (or third) opinion if you find that your difficulties are falling on unsympathetic ears. Early intervention is always better than waiting until you reach crisis point, so don't be afraid to push as much as you feel emotionally able to. Equally, mental health practitioner Mushtag Kahin says, 'If you're not happy with the service, log a complaint.' You should be able to find details of your surgery's complaints policy on their website.

In many areas you may even be able to self-refer for NHS talking therapies through its Improving Access to Psychological Therapies (IAPT) programme, rather than going through your GP (search online for 'IAPT' and your local area). Be aware, though, that availability and waiting times for therapy can be a postcode lottery. In some areas I've heard of patients waiting for years, whereas my own experience has always been closer to weeks or months. Similarly, you may find that the type and quality of mental health support on offer varies.

One of the principles of the IAPT programme is that you should have regular reviews and be allowed a say in your treatment, so don't be afraid to give feedback if something isn't working for you. 'I would say always document your experiences and talk to somebody. Use your voice for change-making, but most importantly make sure to look after yourself, too,' Mushtag says.

For more severe mental health difficulties, having an advocate may also be useful, either in the form of a friend or relative, an independent advocate provided by a charity or other organisation, or a statutory advocate such as an independent mental health advocate (IMHA). See mind.org.uk/information-support/guides -to-support-and-services/advocacy for more details.

Outside the NHS, plenty of charities and activist-led organisations also provide mental health support and signposting, so it's worth searching for services that might be relevant to you, including those listed below. You might also be able to access support in your place of work or education. Mushtag recommends contacting your local Mind or seeking out services specifically tailored to whatever minority communities you're part of.

Resources

In a crisis, call the free, 24/7 Samaritans helpline on **116 123** or the 24/7 National Suicide Prevention Helpline on **0800 689 5652**. If you or someone else needs urgent care, call 999.

General mental health support

- Hub of Hope (search engine for relevant, local support services) – hubofhope.co.uk
- Mind (including local Mind branches in your area) – mind.org.uk or call 0300 123 3393
- SANE – sane.org.uk or call 0300 304 7000 (4.30pm–10.30pm daily)
- Wish (women's mental health) – womenatwish.org.uk or call 020 8980 3618

LGBT+ mental health

- MindOut – mindout.org.uk or call 01273 234839
- Pink Therapy – pinktherapy.com
- Switchboard – switchboard.lgbt or call 0300 330 0630

Black and ethnic minority mental health

- Black Minds Matter UK – blackmindsmatteruk.com
- The Black African and Asian Therapy Network – baatn .org.uk

Support after rape or gendered violence

- Rape Crisis – rapecrisis.org.uk or call 0808 802 9999
- National Domestic Abuse Helpline – nationaldahelpline .org.uk or call 0808 2000 247 (available 24/7)

Neurodiversity

- ADHD Foundation – adhdfoundation.org.uk
- National Autistic Society – autism.org.uk

For a more comprehensive list of support services, see sarah -graham.co.uk/resources-support

6

'Can you get a penis in and a baby out?':
The pleasure gap in sexual health

I started this book by exploring the deeply ingrained sexism and ignorance surrounding long-neglected menstrual health conditions like endometriosis, PMDD and PCOS. Women and others affected by problematic periods too often face gaslighting, dismissive attitudes and gatekeeping about their bodies, and many describe feeling that they are only taken seriously when the issue of fertility and family planning is raised. But in the field of gynaecology these kinds of problems do not begin and end with periods.

In early 2021 I interviewed sexual and reproductive health consultant Dr Janet Barter for an article about the clitoris, and I was particularly struck by one quote that came out of our conversation: 'I really do think that even now, medically speaking, female sexual enjoyment is not seen as important. Too often when gynaecologists – and I can say this because I am one – talk about the vagina, it is purely in terms of "Can you get a penis in and a baby out?"' she said. 'That's all that is ever taught; it's all that's thought about.'

In these few sentences she succinctly summarised what I've so often heard from straight cis women, although I suspect many of them would argue their gynaecologists weren't even particularly worried about the first part. It also, of course, speaks volumes about the issues faced in gynaecology by anyone who isn't interested in getting a penis into their vagina or indeed getting a baby out of it!

As always there are many exceptions to this rule, including the brilliant sexual health professionals who've spoken to me for this chapter, but there are still corners of gynaecology that view vaginas in this simplistic way – as a vessel for male sexual enjoyment and/or procreation. Implicit in this is a lack of concern about female sexual pleasure, which certainly isn't limited to the medical profession.

For a society so obsessed by sex and female sexuality, there's still surprisingly little focus on women's sexual agency and enjoyment. You can see this in what's been dubbed the 'gender orgasm gap': 95% of straight men and 89% of gay men always orgasm during sex, compared to 86% of lesbian women and just 65% of straight women. From sex education to porn and media representations of sex, it's not hard to see where this disparity comes from.

It's been more than half a lifetime since my sex education, but the boys I went to school with were taught about erections and wet dreams from about the age of 10. They grew up doodling cocks and balls, expecting pleasure, and viewing themselves as the dominant players in sexual conquest. As girls, our sex education focused mostly on the mechanics of avoiding pregnancy.

The sex positive movement has come a long way since then, but women are still too often viewed as passive recipients – the people who sex happens to – and the female orgasm framed as incidental, or even mysterious and mythical. While male masturbation is talked and joked about as a fact of life, female masturbation remains far more taboo and shrouded in shame – keeping many women totally unaware of their clitoris until well into adult life.

This ignorance of our anatomy is a problem, both in terms of sexual pleasure, but also vulval and vaginal health more broadly. In 2014, research by gynaecological cancer charity the Eve

Appeal found that 44% of women couldn't identify the vagina (internal genitalia) on a diagram, while 60% didn't know what the vulva (external genitalia) was.

Perhaps more depressingly, a 2013 review of medical textbooks found a distinct lack of accurate information about normal, healthy female genitalia. It's also worth noting that although the detailed anatomy of the clitoris was first depicted in the 19th century, it wasn't until 2005 that this information became more widely known, thanks to the work of Australian urologist Helen O'Connell. It, too, is still notably absent from many medical textbooks.

Likewise, medical research has hugely prioritised issues like erectile dysfunction over female sexual problems. The same is very much true when it comes to clinical practice and treatment options. More recent research by the Eve Appeal found that cis women are nearly five times as likely as cis men to feel not listened to by a healthcare professional when seeking help for a reproductive health issue. Women were also twice as likely as men to leave the appointment feeling like they'd raised a 'trivial' issue.

The field of sexual health is also awash with intersectional biases. Women of colour, women with physical and learning disabilities, and queer, trans and non-binary people are all on the receiving end of biased assumptions about their sexual health needs. For disabled journalist Lucy Webster, who uses a wheelchair, a major source of frustration is doctors speaking to her like a child and automatically assuming she's not sexually active. 'The first time I went to the doctor about going on the pill, I was 19 and at university, and she said, "I assume it's just to control your periods." That was all I wanted it for at the time – because having a period when you're disabled is a bloody nightmare – but I hated the assumption that I didn't need it for contraception as well,' Lucy says.

Likewise, 'There are a lot of assumptions about Black people's intellect and ability to make decisions or understand,' says Dr Annabel Sowemimo, a community sexual and reproductive health doctor and founder of Decolonising Contraception, an organisation set up to support the sexual and reproductive health of Black people and people of colour. 'Black patients often feel talked down to, given a lesser explanation or just told what's going to happen to them.'

When you put all these factors together, sexual and reproductive healthcare can be a minefield for anyone born with a vagina. In reproductive-age cis women, the prevalence of female sexual dysfunction (FSD) is estimated at 41% worldwide. Equally, gynaecological and urogynaecological issues like lichen sclerosus, pudendal neuralgia, chronic urinary tract infections (UTIs) and vulvodynia can take a toll outside the bedroom, seeping into the much broader contexts of sufferers' everyday lives. And then there's the enormous burden of contraception and fertility, which, in cis heterosexual relationships, falls overwhelmingly to women.

*

FSD is an umbrella term used to describe a whole range of issues, from problems with libido, arousal or orgasm to painful sex (dyspareunia). Despite the name, the various forms of FSD can affect anyone with a vagina, but these conditions are typically hampered by the same sexist assumptions and attitudes we've seen elsewhere – namely, that everyone with a vagina is cis, heterosexual, not that interested in sex anyway and should just find other ways to 'please their man'. One woman, whose vaginal pain had left her unable to enjoy intimacy with her husband, told me her doctor had helpfully responded with, 'There are plenty of ways to skin a cat.' Others tell me repeatedly about doctors wheeling out stock phrases like, 'Have a glass of wine,' 'Lie back and think of England,' or 'Just try to relax.'

Lack of medical knowledge and understanding is, naturally, a huge part of this. 'I came out of medical school in 2003 and I was never taught the anatomy of the clitoris. It just never came up. Even in my sexual health registrar training, it never cropped up. There was nothing on clitoral stimulation or how a woman orgasms,' says Dr Naomi Sutton, a consultant in sexual health and TV doctor for Channel 4's *The Sex Clinic*. 'When I first did *The Sex Clinic* I felt completely unarmed to talk about female pleasure and sexual dysfunction. Things may have changed since I was trained, but we definitely need to do better and have more of a focus on female pleasure in gynae and sexual health services,' she adds.

Equally though, Naomi says: '[Doctors] are subject to the same social and cultural pressures as everybody else; just because we're medics doesn't mean we've not got hang-ups about sex. I don't think we get enough training in how to talk about it, which can be really difficult. Some people are naturals, but for other doctors it's awkward as hell.'

Fran Bushe, author of *My Broken Vagina*, tells me she heard very similar things from the doctors she interviewed, with a combination of embarrassment and lack of knowledge being key contributors to the difficulties women face when seeking healthcare for sexual dysfunction or pain. In addition to this, though, there also seems to be an underlying attitude that sexual pleasure isn't really a medical problem; that women's ability to have an enjoyable sex life is beyond doctors' remit. 'There does seem to be this mindset that enjoying sex isn't really important and that it's all in your head,' she says.

There's a double irony in this. Psychosexual therapy – one of the few treatment options recommended for a range of female sexual issues, which addresses the psychological issues believed to underlie some types of FSD – is rarely covered on the NHS. 'The way healthcare is now commissioned means psychosexual services typically fall through the cracks,' Dr Janet Barter explains. 'Sexual health, including contraception and STI [sexually transmitted infection] testing, is funded by local authorities. Most other healthcare, including gynaecology, is funded by clinical commissioning groups [now known as integrated care boards]. What happened with psychosexual work was that it didn't fall into either camp, so it's not funded as part of gynaecology and it's not funded as part of sexual health.'

In some areas, including the one where Janet works, clinicians have successfully fought for joint funding. However, as Hysterical Women contributor Helen (not her real name) discovered, psychosexual therapy is not covered in most areas. When she presented to her university surgery with anorgasmia (inability to reach orgasm), she was pleasantly surprised to find her GP both attentive and sympathetic. However, after Helen had detailed her 'colourful mental health history' her GP concluded the cause was probably psychological. 'As such, I was not offered any kind of physical examination or tests. I was advised to seek psychosexual therapy, but told that this was not offered by the local NHS trust – i.e. I would need to pay for it myself,' Helen writes. 'I wonder how the doctor would have responded to my anorgasmia if I was a 21-year-old cis man. Would a physical investigation have been deemed unnecessary? Would I have been advised to make room in my student budget for private therapy? I somehow doubt it,' she adds.

This isn't to say that psychological factors can't or don't play a role. Women are more likely than men to have suffered previous sexual trauma, which can contribute to painful conditions like vaginismus – an involuntary tightening of the muscles around the vagina whenever penetration is attempted. Similarly, previous experiences of painful sex can trigger a vicious cycle of anxiety, tension and more pain for many sufferers. Psychological factors such as poor mental health, stress, relationship dissatisfaction and religious beliefs are all recognised as 'significant risk factors' of FSD, but so too are physical factors, including poor physical health, genitourinary problems and female genital mutilation (FGM). Hormonal deficiencies may also play a role, as can underlying conditions like diabetes or depression, and certain medications – including, ironically, antidepressants and hormonal contraceptives. To dismiss these complex issues as purely psychological is hugely problematic, feeding yet again into the same old sexist ideas about women's bodies and sexualities.

Janet believes the optimum solution would be to treat female sexual problems holistically, but this can only happen when joint services are properly funded. Her service uses a combined clinic between a doctor and a psychologist. 'We can look at the psychological side of things, but we can also look to see if there is a skin problem, an anatomical problem or a hormonal issue,' she explains. Vaginismus, for example, can be treated using a combination of psychosexual therapy and relaxation exercises – to break the vicious cycle of fear and pain – alongside pelvic floor physiotherapy and dilation, where tampon-shaped plastic tubes, in increasing sizes, are used to gently stretch the vagina and get it used to penetration.

Currently, though, patient experiences of seeking help for vaginismus are a real mixed bag, according to Lisa Mackenzie, founder of the Vaginismus Network. 'Imagine if someone builds up the courage to speak to their GP about something that is so incredibly personal and they're told to just have a glass of wine to relax; that it's not an issue,' she says. 'This could set their progress back by months or even years. They may trust what they're told by the professional person in a position of power, rather than challenge and persevere for the right answer, and [as a result of this treatment] may end up not addressing the issue again for some time. I've also heard from people who knew the advice they were being given wasn't quite right, but the flippant nature of it knocked their confidence or made them feel silly for going to their GP in the first place.'

That said, Lisa doesn't believe we can lay all the blame or responsibility on GPs. 'If conditions like vaginismus were prioritised and funded at an earlier stage, I believe there's more chance it would be taken seriously by GPs,' she says. Indeed, according to Cynthia Graham, Professor of Sexual and Reproductive Health, in many cases it's not that there's a lack of research into female sexual dysfunction. She believes the main issue is partly that this knowledge doesn't filter down into medical training and education, and partly – as Janet says – that there often aren't relevant services available for GPs to refer patients on to.

*

While vaginismus is triggered by penetration, there are also several vulval and vaginal conditions characterised by more persistent pain and discomfort. Georgia (not her real name) has suffered from a chronic inflammatory vulval skin condition called lichen sclerosus since she was just nine years old, when she would clutch bags of frozen peas to her crotch to numb the incessant itching. Lichen sclerosus – which can affect the vulva, vagina, anus or penis, but is significantly more common in women – causes patches of skin to become itchy, sore, cracked and inflamed, eventually leaving it tight and scarred and, if left untreated, increasing the risk of vulval or penile cancer.

Georgia was in her early 20s, and finding sex with her long-term partner less and less appealing, by the time she got a diagnosis. The 'unsympathetic, pervy male doctor' who diagnosed her had stared at her breasts throughout the consultation so, when the steroid cream he'd prescribed didn't work, she asked to be referred to a different dermatologist. This subsequent appointment was with a woman, who Georgia hoped would be more understanding. Instead, she dismissed Georgia's pain as 'psychological', writing her off as an 'anxious person' for expressing concern about potential damage to her labia and prescribing the same steroid cream she'd already tried. A subsequent doctor offered the unsolicited advice that she should simply have more sex with her partner to improve her symptoms.

By January 2020 Georgia's symptoms were unbearable. She was constantly itching, struggling to sleep, have sex or concentrate on uni work, and having daily breakdowns. Desperate, she sought out a lichen sclerosus specialist, who told her the steroid she'd been using for years was incorrect, before prescribing a long list of creams, to be used daily, and a far more potent steroid cream to manage her symptoms. It took months of this intensive treatment to get her symptoms under control and Georgia has since learned that her experience is 'not an uncommon one for women with lichen sclerosus. I'm still often told by doctors that I am "too young" to have lichen sclerosus, and my diagnosis and personal experiences are routinely questioned,' she says. 'I have suffered so much unnecessary pain, simply because I am a woman with an under-researched, underfunded and often undiagnosed disorder.'

When Marion Jones' chronic pelvic and vulval pain was dismissed by a consultant gynaecologist as 'all psychological', it sparked a fire in her. An unlikely activist, the former NHS worker has since dedicated her life to raising awareness and campaigning for better treatment of women like her. Marion suffers from pudendal neuralgia (chronic pelvic pain caused by damage to the pudendal nerve) and vulvodynia (persistent and unexplained vulval pain) – both of which, in her case, were triggered by prolapse surgery. Marion's pain is constant, robbing her of her ability to work, socialise and even sit down for more than 15 minutes at a time.

After co-founding a Facebook support group for UK sufferers of pudendal neuralgia – now more than 1100 members strong – Marion learned that she was far from the only woman to have had her pain dismissed as psychological or 'all in your head'. As well as raising awareness through both traditional and social media, Marion has gone on to produce information leaflets for patients and healthcare professionals, met with her local hospital PALS (the organisation that supports NHS patients) and lobbied her local MP for support. 'I had suffered more than enough pain in the previous eight years and there was no way I was going to accept what [the consultant] had said,' she writes on Hysterical Women. 'Friends and family who had been there for me all the way through could see the pain written on my face every day. All I want now is for this never to happen to any other woman again,' she adds.

Fellow vulvodynia sufferer Claire's (not her real name) symptoms came on 'almost overnight' when she was just 19 years old. Having previously had 'perfectly comfortable and pain-free intercourse', suddenly she found herself unable to have sex, ride her bike or sit down for long periods without a burning, stinging or aching sensation in her vulva. Despite this, a gynaecologist informed Claire that she was 'perfectly healthy', with nothing visibly wrong, and advised her to pay for psychosexual counselling. Claire was immediately sceptical: 'My symptoms had begun during a healthy and happy relationship, I had no history of trauma, my pain was not just related to sexual or medical penetration, and the burning sensation was particularly pronounced on one side of the vestibule,' she says. 'But the gynaecologist repeated that things "down there" were complicated, and I was willing to accept that the interconnection between body and mind was beyond my comprehension. But more importantly, I was desperate.'

As she'd expected, Claire's expensive, self-funded therapy didn't help and she now firmly believes that 'For someone with my symptoms and history, this should not have been the first and only treatment option that was explored.' It wasn't until several years later that she stumbled across an article on vulvodynia that provided her with the answers she'd been looking for. 'Having a name for my condition was validating and empowering,' she says. Unfortunately, though, she quickly discovered that vulvodynia is poorly understood and under-researched.

Claire's experience inspired her to launch Lip Service, a not-for-profit zine that aims to shine a light on the experiences and projects of pelvic pain sufferers, through interviews, articles, poetry, collage and art. Through her own research, she also found and requested a referral to a specialist research centre, where a dermatologist reassured her that her pain was real and diagnosed provoked vulvodynia five years after the onset of her symptoms. According to vulvodynia researcher Claudia Chisari this is fairly typical. 'Many women don't get diagnosed for a very long time. Research shows women typically see at least three doctors before they get a diagnosis of vulvodynia and 40% never get a diagnosis,' she says.

From Claudia's perspective, a common problem is one of misdiagnosis and over-medicalisation, where doctors prescribe treatments that either mask or actually worsen the symptoms. 'With vulvodynia there's no damage to the skin, there's no infection, but doctors often end up prescribing antibiotics. That then causes thrush, which inflames the area and makes things even worse,' she explains. In an ideal world, she adds, diagnosis would happen much quicker – as soon as sexually transmitted infections (STIs) and cancer have been ruled out – and the first-line treatment would be pelvic physiotherapy, allowing patients to take ownership of their health through pelvic floor exercises and dilation, instead of relying on medications.

In the meantime, her research project at King's College London proposes a biopsychosocial model, using acceptance and commitment therapy (ACT) to address the psychological toll of living with vulvodynia. This model, she says, acknowledges how vulvodynia symptoms affect women's everyday lives, from work to socialising and relationships. 'If vulvodynia was recognised and diagnosed earlier, the psychosocial impact would be much less. But currently there's a lot of invalidation surrounding the diagnosis, where women are not understood or believed. This invalidation, in a way, is more painful than the actual symptoms – there's no recognition of how the symptoms interfere with their lives,' she explains.

*

This kind of invalidation is also common for women affected by chronic urinary tract infections (UTIs). More than 80% of people affected by UTIs are women, with 50–60% of all women likely to develop at least one in their lifetime. Symptoms include pain or a burning sensation when peeing, needing to pee more frequently, and cloudy or bloody pee. Although they can be diagnosed based on symptoms alone, UTIs are typically diagnosed, regardless of symptoms, by referring to a urine culture. This test, in use since the 1950s, has long been considered the gold standard. The other technique commonly used is a dipstick test, which may detect the presence of white blood cells in the urine. The problem is that neither test is accurate enough for the role they play. As Milly Storr discovered after years of recurrent infections, this reliance on urine testing can result in patients being dismissed if their samples come back negative.

Like many women, Milly got her first UTI after becoming sexually active, at the age of 16. The infection lasted an agonising six months, causing her to miss a lot of school – but Milly's family GP dismissed it as 'honeymoon cystitis', prescribed a short course of antibiotics and left her to get on with it. Her next serious UTI came during her first year at university. 'Sex is a really common trigger for UTIs and for me it was typically when I changed partners. I'd just got into a new relationship and ended up being really unwell for a very long time,' Milly explains. This time the infection lasted nine months and resulted in her being hospitalised after she started peeing a lot of blood.

But Milly's issues really started with her third UTI, the following year, when her dipstick test came back negative. Despite having the same symptoms and seeing the same doctor, Milly suddenly found herself refused treatment. 'The doctor said it was negative, so I didn't have a UTI. I was like, "I definitely do. I can feel it, I promise you," but she insisted there was nothing she could give me,' she recalls. This went on for several months, during which time Milly again became so ill she could barely get out of bed – except to go to the toilet every five minutes.

After her illness forced her to drop out of uni, Milly paid to see a private urogynaecologist, who had the exact same response: 'There's nothing wrong with you.' It was only when Milly stumbled across a newspaper article about the work of the late Professor James Malone-Lee, a specialist in urinary infections, that she began finding some answers.

Before his death in 2022, James – an Emeritus Professor of Medicine at University College London and author of *Cystitis Unmasked* – told me: 'These tests were based on the assumption that the normal bladder was sterile – and that was wrong. A lot of aspects of medicine have not been tested properly, and there's a long history of our profession working on assumptions and presumptions. The urine test wasn't remotely properly validated, but it became the gold standard.'

Indeed, research published in 2018 confirmed that the urine culture test is 'not fit for purpose' and 'spectacularly' fails to diagnose most sufferers of chronic UTIs. Despite this, many doctors have continued to rely on both urine cultures and dipstick tests for a definitive diagnosis, gaslighting patients like Milly whose results come back negative.

There is some hope on the horizon for those living with chronic UTIs though. As recently as March 2022, in response to pressure from campaigners, the NHS updated its online patient information to include chronic UTIs for the first time. 'In some people, antibiotics do not work or urine tests do not pick up an infection, even though you have UTI symptoms,' the update states. 'This may mean you have a long-term (chronic) UTI that is not picked up by current urine tests. Ask the GP for a referral to a specialist for further tests and treatments.'

It will no doubt take time for this information to filter through into GPs' training and practice, but for campaigners it's an important first step – an acknowledgement of their experiences, and an authoritative proof to present to their doctors. It's also another example of the power of patient activism and advocacy which will, I'm sure, benefit so many future generations of patients. In the meantime though, experiences like Milly's highlight bigger issues about how healthcare's knowledge gap and trust gap interact, and the devastation this can cause.

James believed modern medicine's obsession with tests often leads doctors into a 'base rate fallacy', where they place too much emphasis on test results at the expense of all the other evidence in front of them. 'If you come to me and describe all the signs and symptoms of a UTI, the probability that you have a UTI is quite high. I might ask you some questions, your responses to which cause that probability to be even higher. Then I might press on your abdomen and, if it hurts, the probability is higher still. But then someone does a urine culture and announces, "Oh, there's no urine infection. It's negative." That is a massive scientific clanger, because you ignore the base-rate probability prior to the test,' he said.

The impact of this on patients – most of them women – has been enormous, James added. 'There's a huge variation, but it takes an average of six and a half years of suffering before women get to my clinic. In the NHS clinic I used to run, the average is now 11 years. And their lives are ruined,' he explained. 'They commonly can't work, they can't socially interact. They're ill and in pain an awful lot of the time. They can't have sex and their relationship might have come to an end as a result. It's calamitous, an awful mess.'

So often I find myself wondering how on earth any doctor could send women away in this kind of state. But, like most of the issues we've explored so far, it's complex. 'You've got a profession that's hidebound to positive/negative tests. You then have the fact that if people have been taught that something is true, it takes an awful lot of work to get them to think differently,' James says. 'The other thing is, when you're confronted by this new information, you have to address the fact that, looking back over your history, you've told many, many patients – predominantly women – there was nothing wrong with them. And you were wrong and they were right. That's a hell of an undertaking, so you're going to meet an enormous amount of cognitive dissonance,' he adds.

Beyond diagnostics, there's also an issue around how chronic UTIs are treated. While many UTIs clear up after a single, short course of antibiotics, around 30% don't. The professor's approach to chronic UTIs was to use longer-term courses of antibiotics until the symptoms completely clear. This has proved controversial, particularly in the context of concerns around antibiotic resistance. But, again, the research proves it works. A review of 624 patient outcomes by the Lower Urinary Tract Symptoms clinic in Hornsey, north London, found that almost all the women treated in this way got better, just one had a serious side-effect and there was no evidence of antimicrobial resistance.

For Milly, long-term antibiotic treatment has been life-changing, allowing her to return to university and complete her psychology degree. Her dissertation subject was stigma and delegitimisation in chronic pain patients, and she now hopes to attend medical school to train as a specialist in the treatment of biofilm infections (biofilms are thin layers of bacterial cells, often involved in UTIs). 'I'm just so fed up with the system,' she says. 'The NHS needs a huge shake-up because the treatment of women with chronic infections is diabolical. It's the most frustrating thing in the whole world not to be listened to when you're so unwell.'

*

We cannot, of course, talk about the treatment of vulvas and vaginas without discussing the single biggest women's health scandal of the 21st century: vaginal and pelvic mesh. The most common vaginal mesh is the tension-free vaginal tape (TVT), a plastic implant made from polypropylene, similar to those still used in hernia repairs and bowel surgery. It was sold as a 'quick fix' to common problems like urinary incontinence and prolapse, but, for many women, their 'quick fix' became a nightmare.

Looking back, Kath Sansom says, the incontinence she sought help for really wasn't that bad. A mother of two daughters, Kath had taken up boxing after her marriage ended and experienced the kind of mild leaking that many women – particularly mothers – struggle with later in life. 'I would just leak a bit when I was exercising or if I did a few sneezes in a row. It wasn't even a full-on leak, it was just an annoyance,' she says.

Instead of being referred for pelvic physiotherapy, which Kath now knows would likely have solved her issues, she was advised to have a mesh implant. 'I was told it was a really simple solution and I honestly thought it would just be like having a coil fitted. They called it a 'sling', not a mesh. I wasn't even told that it was plastic or that it was permanent. That procedure completely ruined my life and my health, all for a bit of leaking,' she tells me.

After having the mesh fitted in March 2015, Kath experienced instant pain and regret. 'I immediately felt that I'd made the worst decision of my life. I just knew something was really wrong and I needed to get this thing out,' she says. Despite this, her surgeon downplayed Kath's symptoms, insisting things would settle down and that they'd never had any problems before. 'Right from the word go I was treated like a mystery patient. It was so belittling and they obviously just wanted to make me go away,' she adds.

Frustrated, Kath turned to Google. 'There wasn't much out there at the time, but I started seeing the word "complications" and I connected with a woman in Oxford who'd had a similar experience,' she says. Within three weeks of having surgery, Kath had begun interviewing other women and making plans to launch a campaign: Sling the Mesh.

With a Facebook support group now 9000 members strong, Sling the Mesh has been hugely influential in shining a light on women's experiences, transforming attitudes towards the use of mesh and lobbying for policy change. 'The common themes I hear about over and over again are women being ignored, being made to feel stupid, or that they're weak for not coping, and doctors blaming their symptoms on something else. There has been institutional denial,' Kath says.

In reality, she says, symptoms most commonly include pain in the vagina, legs and lower back, urinary tract infections and loss of sex life. 'I should say,' she adds, 'my GP was amazing when

I did go to him. He got me the referral to go in for my mesh removal. Not once did he ever question why I was there or make me feel stupid, not once did he refuse me the pain relief I needed to make my life better. From that respect I have been so lucky, especially as the mesh removal did save my sex life. For some people, even after removal, their sex life is ruined because of permanent nerve damage.'

Kath launched Sling the Mesh in June 2015, just months after her surgery, driven by a 'strong conviction and sense of duty, as a woman and a journalist'. It's no exaggeration to say that she has since proven herself to be one of the most formidable campaigners of her generation. Over the following few years, Kath's sustained media and social media campaign saw the issue covered by Sky News, the *Daily Mail*, *Victoria Derbyshire* and many more. 'It really was breaking down a lot of taboos at the time – talking about vaginas, incontinence, the loss of people's sex lives,' she says.

Widespread media coverage lent the campaign sufficient weight for Kath to take her message to the Houses of Parliament, with Sling the Mesh holding their first rally in 2017 and encouraging supporters to write to their MPs. 'Honestly, I don't think anyone knows how much time I put into this other than my daughters and best friends. For six years, constantly, I'd be up until midnight, then up again at 4 o'clock in the morning, emailing politicians, emailing people in the NHS, or geeing up the group to tweet, or join a rally, or write to their MP,' she says. 'Sometimes I'd have to just escape to my beach hut in Norfolk and have a cry by the sea. It weighs on me really heavily and I've had to learn how to look after my own wellbeing. You can't fight if you're stressed, exhausted and burnt out.'

By 2018, Kath's blood, sweat and tears were finally beginning to pay off. Vaginal mesh surgery was suspended on the NHS as a treatment for incontinence and then health secretary Jeremy Hunt announced the Cumberlege Review, which would investigate three major women's health scandals, including the injuries caused by pelvic mesh. Baroness Julia Cumberlege spent two and a half years hearing evidence of women's experiences. When her report, *First Do No Harm*, was published in July 2020, it was damning. Not only had thousands of women suffered avoidable harm, but many of those same women had repeatedly been ignored and let down; their life-changing symptoms dismissed as 'women's problems'.

For Kath, the battle is far from over. A year on from the report's publication, she tells me that all the Government has done for mesh-injured women so far is 'a half-hearted apology from [then health secretary] Matt Hancock'. The Government has already ruled out offering financial redress to victims, which was one of the nine recommendations made in the report. In 2022 Dr Henrietta Hughes OBE was appointed as the UK's first Patient Safety Commissioner – a role created in response to those recommendations. However, the remaining recommendations, including specialist treatment centres for those affected, are yet to be fully implemented.

Despite this, Kath says, 'I do feel very proud of my legacy. I'm particularly proud of the broader women's health movement that's emerged off the back of the mesh campaign, in terms of highlighting medical misogyny and gaslighting. The Cumberlege Review proves these are real issues, and I hope we've inspired women to go off and do their own research, so they can speak to their doctors in a more informed way.' Finally, I ask, does she have any parting advice for patient advocates and campaigners? 'Don't let the bastards grind you down,' she says with a defiant grin.

*

While women's pleasure and even comfort are too often not prioritised, we are still expected to take responsibility for preventing unwanted pregnancies. In the majority of heterosexual relationships, the 'admin' of contraception – from deciding what to use, to making the appointments, collecting the prescriptions and going for the check-ups – still invariably falls to the woman. The 2021 announcement that men under 25 would no longer be routinely offered chlamydia screening, while women the same age would, simply reinforced the message that sexual health is a woman's problem. Heterosexual men, it appears, are entirely free from responsibility when it comes to their sexual exploits, despite being fertile every day of the month, compared to women's (approximately) six-day fertile window.

There's no doubt that access to contraception, which is freely available on the NHS, is a big deal. The development of the contraceptive pill during the late 1960s and early 1970s was a landmark moment for feminism. The pill and its more recent siblings – the coil, implant, injection, etc. – continue to be vital tools for women's liberation, allowing us to choose when, and if, we want to have children. But is it enough to simply protect women from unwanted pregnancies or, as we've explored in other areas of medicine, do sexual healthcare professionals need to start considering our quality of life as well?

Certainly, a lack of innovation and concerns about contraceptive side-effects have left a growing number of women feeling dissatisfied and even anxious about the choices available to them in recent years. Inspired by her own struggle to find a solution that worked for her, in 2019 Alice Pelton launched The Lowdown. Described as a 'Tripadvisor for contraception', it provides user-generated ratings and reviews of all the forms of contraception currently available in the UK, allowing women to access a concise overview of the side-effects, pros and cons of each option.

In 2017 journalist Vicky Spratt launched an investigation into the mental health side-effects of the contraceptive pill. This investigation, Mad About the Pill, was fuelled by readers' stories, but also inspired by her own experience. 'I had suffered with hormonal contraception for years and at one point had a complete mental breakdown whilst on the progestogen-only pill,' she tells me. 'I had terrible treatment from GPs, being fobbed off and prescribed antidepressants and beta blockers. I ended up having a really, really scary experience where I was having suicidal thoughts, which I'd never experienced before in my life.'

When Vicky started looking into this, she learned there's clear evidence within the medical community that the hormones in the pill can, in some women, cause depression and anxiety. Despite this, she says, 'The NHS website and leaflets at the time listed side-effects as including "mood changes" – well, that's not the same as having suicidal thoughts or severe anxiety that's so bad you can't leave the house.'

As for why these and other side-effects occur, and who's most likely to be susceptible, 'This is still an area there's not much research on,' Professor Cynthia Graham tells me. In her own research, Cynthia has focused on sexual side-effects of the contraceptive pill, but, she says, 'Lack of funding is a major issue. Of all the topics I've worked on, it's not the one that gets funding.'

What we do know, Cynthia explains, is that there's a subgroup of women who experience negative sexual side-effects, like changes to libido. 'What we don't know – and I would have loved to research this – is what the predictors of that are,' she adds. 'There aren't any studies looking at whether some specific formulations of pills are more likely to lead to sexual negative side-effects. As a result, there's still no basis on which to say to a woman who's having side-effects, "This pill would be good for you to try instead." It's trial and error. The same is absolutely true with mental health side-effects.'

The rollout of the UK's Covid-19 vaccination programme in 2021 also reignited conversations about the (small) blood clot risk associated with the pill, after concerns were raised about links between the AstraZeneca vaccine and a very small number of rare blood clots in younger vaccine recipients. Many sexual health services pointed out that both risks were incredibly low (0.05%–01.2% for the combined pill and 0.0004% for the vaccine), particularly compared to the much higher blood clot risks associated with both pregnancy and contracting Covid-19. However, conversations online pondered why the vaccine risks had been taken so seriously so quickly, with all under 40s offered alternative jabs, when women have been expected to live with the risks associated with the pill for decades.

Similar discontent was expressed in 2016, when trials of a long-awaited and potentially ground-breaking male contraceptive were stopped early after male participants encountered negative side-effects, including depression, acne and changes to libido. These side-effects, as many people pointed out, were strikingly similar to those that had long been deemed an acceptable price for women to pay for the avoidance of unwanted pregnancies. 'There's a gender bias there for sure and I don't think it's just that men are more intolerant of the side-effects,' Cynthia says. 'I think doctors, and maybe some researchers, think it's less important when the effects are on women.'

*

Of course, for many women the pill continues to be the game-changer it was originally conceived as. My own experience, after a bit of trial and error to find a brand that worked for me, was overwhelmingly positive. I took the pill for a decade with minimal concerns or complaints except the very long time it took for my cycle to regulate again afterwards. From all the women I've spoken to about this over the years, it's clear that there's no one size fits all when it comes to contraception. And, while Alice believes there's always some kind of trade-off, different women will have different priorities when making their choice.

'The pill and hormonal methods all have similar clusters of side-effects that affect some women more than others, and different women care about different things – skin, sex drive, mood and so on. Some women hate hormonal options so much that their tolerance of the bleeding, pain and heavy periods that can come with the non-hormonal copper IUD is much higher. They're just so happy to not be getting pregnant or dealing with hormonal side-effects,' Alice explains. 'I often think it also depends on what you've tried before and how you've come to this method. Even though my periods were very painful with the

IUD, I'd previously felt very depressed on the pill and so I was very happy to have excruciating periods as the alternative.'

Certainly, Alice adds, The Lowdown hears from a lot of people who are desperate for new non-hormonal methods. But, she says, there's been so little innovation and funding in this area for so long that women seeking non-hormonal alternatives are currently left with either the copper IUD, the fertility awareness method (including cycle and fertility tracking apps like Natural Cycles) or just using condoms. Both of the latter are particularly susceptible to user error. Condoms are 98% effective with perfect use, but only 82% effective with typical use. Meanwhile, fertility awareness methods – while extremely effective with perfect use – have an estimated 76-88% efficacy with typical use and can't be relied on if you have an irregular cycle.

The IUD, too, is not without its issues, with some women experiencing agonising pain during and after having one fitted. Lucy Cohen was inspired by her own experience to launch a petition calling for better pain relief to be provided for IUD insertions and removals, prompting media figures like Naga Munchetty and Caitlin Moran to share their own stories of painful IUD fittings.

After suffering arterial blood clots in 2021, Lucy was told she could no longer use hormonal contraception. 'The IUD was a really good solution for me – it lasts for 10 years, once it's in it's in, so that was what I opted for,' she tells me. Having heard the fitting could be painful, Lucy requested pain relief beforehand, but was reassured that paracetamol should be fine. In reality, she says, her experience was 'absolutely horrific'. 'It was excruciatingly painful, to the point where I didn't recognise the sounds coming out of my mouth. It took three attempts to measure and fit it, and I just wasn't prepared for the experience at all,' Lucy says.

Traumatised by what had happened, Lucy started asking other women about their experiences – just friends at first, then a survey which she shared on Twitter – and found that she wasn't alone. 'It's still open, but I've had about 1500 responses so far and the stories are heart-breaking. Obviously, it's self-selecting, but 71%

of people said they were not prepared and didn't feel adequately informed about what the procedure was, and 95% of people said there should be better pain relief,' Lucy says.

'There's a massive issue here about consent, because they talk you through all the risks, but when it comes to pain, the NHS website says some women may experience "discomfort". Discomfort is what you experience when you get your eyebrows threaded; I never consented to be in as much pain as I was in, so it feels like a violation,' she adds. Her petition called for better expectation management and more pain relief options to be offered as standard, so that all patients opting for an IUD can give truly informed consent. 'To my mind this is quite an easily solvable problem. Just listen to women and treat putting things into their uteruses with the same gravitas that we treat non-gendered procedures like colonoscopies,' Lucy says.

In response to Lucy's campaign, the Faculty of Sexual and Reproductive Healthcare (FSRH), which sets professional standards of care for sexual health doctors in the UK, has now updated its guidance to recommend that all women should be offered pain relief for coil fittings. Across the sexual health sector, though, responses to Lucy's campaign varied, from the defensive and dismissive 'It shouldn't hurt' to those calling for a more open dialogue. The same has been true in conversations about side-effects of the pill and other hormonal contraceptives. In submissions to #ShitMyDoctorSays, numerous women have described doctors flat out refusing to accept the side-effects they've experienced. Others have experienced the kind of shrugging it off attitude that this is simply the price you have to pay for not getting pregnant.

We also need to talk about the issue of contraceptive coercion, which Dr Annabel Sowemimo says is a problem Decolonising Contraception sees, particularly with younger and racially minoritised patients. 'We hear a lot from people who've said they want a particular [long-acting] contraceptive removed, but they're told "Just wait a bit longer" or "I don't think that's the right thing to do." There might be a good reason for that, which should be explained, like if they're more likely to have a high-risk pregnancy, but ultimately you have to respect a patient's autonomy,' she says.

A 2021 report by the British Pregnancy Advisory Service found that certain groups experience pressure to accept long-acting reversible contraceptive methods, like a coil, implant or injection – including Black and women of colour, those with higher BMIs and those with physical or mental health issues. Black and women of colour faced racist stereotypes about promiscuity and young parenthood, as well as racial bias in pain assessment. Meanwhile, disabled people and those with mental health issues often felt their autonomy was undermined, with healthcare professionals assuming they 'knew best.'

For some doctors, there are understandable concerns that talking about risks or side-effects may increase patients' anxiety, putting them off using safe, effective forms of contraception. They fear this will lead to women discontinuing contraception altogether and a rise in unintended pregnancies – like the mid-90s 'pill panic', which saw a 25% increase in births and a 9% increase in abortion rates following widespread media coverage of studies into blood clot risk. In my view, though, refusing to acknowledge women's experiences and concerns also serves to deepen the mistrust. Instead, we desperately need doctors to engage with patients as adults, in an honest and realistic way, so they can make informed choices about all the currently available options.

'Very rarely women will react really badly to a coil fitting, but for the vast majority of women who have a coil fitted it's a very short-lived amount of pain,' Dr Naomi Sutton tells me. 'Most of the evidence shows that the biggest factor is who's fitting it – if you've got someone confident and well-trained fitting it, and the patient feels comfortable and relaxed, it's much more likely to go well. I do worry that these kinds of stories will heighten patients' anxiety and make them more tense, when actually the majority of women don't suffer this kind of pain when they have a coil fitted and, for lots of people, it's an absolutely amazing option,' she explains.

That said, Naomi adds, she's always clear with patients from the off that it's their body and they're in control. 'I definitely wouldn't carry on if someone was screaming on the bed, because, even if they haven't said "No" or "Stop" that's them withdrawing their consent, just like when you're having sex. We can't assault a patient; we have to be honest and have an open dialogue. If someone can't tolerate the coil, we'd look at something else. There is always something for everybody,' she says.

YOUR SEXUAL AND GYNAE HEALTH TOOLKIT

Let's be honest, seeking healthcare for sexual and gynae issues is never going to be the most comfortable situation for most of us. When you combine that with cuts to services – or even a total lack of services in some cases – there's no denying it can be really difficult to access the care you need, whether that's for contraception, sexual issues or more general vulval and vaginal pain.

However, there are ways you can improve your chances and the first tip I always give is to check out the list of staff on your GP surgery's website. This page will list each GP's special interests and additional training, and you may find that one of them specialises in sexual health. If so, try to book an appointment with that GP – they'll likely be the most comfortable talking about these issues, as well as being most clued up on the latest research. Alternatively, doctors and nurses at specialist sexual health clinics will be much more used to talking about these issues all day long – you can find your nearest by clicking 'Sexual health services' at nhs.uk/nhs-services.

From there, as we've seen elsewhere, it's mostly a question of doing your research and going in with clear expectations. 'One of the ways patients can get what they want out of a consultation is by bringing a list of questions. Let your doctor know at the start of the consultation that you're in the driving seat. It's not about undermining their authority and you should have confidence in your doctor, but by coming in, explaining what's happened already and asking to share your list of questions, you establish your own authority. What is your key concern? What are your expectations?' says sexual and reproductive health doctor Annabel Sowemimo.

'Some doctors actually appreciate this because it provides some clarity and I do believe most of my colleagues want their patients to do well,' she adds. 'If you're nervous or wary about medical institutions, having these things written down also helps you remember to cover everything you wanted to talk about.'

For complex or chronic issues, which your GP may be less well-informed about, it's always worth checking out relevant charities and peer support groups for advice and information before your consultation. Living with vulval or vaginal pain can be incredibly isolating to deal with on your own, but there is support available, as well as signposting to relevant specialists and resources.

Similarly, seeking out other people's experiences of different contraceptive methods can help you to make a more informed choice about what might work best for you. There's still an element of trial and error involved – what works like a dream for your best friend could turn out to be your worst nightmare – but sites like The Lowdown can at least provide a more comprehensive overview of the pros and cons. As I've mentioned elsewhere, keeping a diary of your symptoms or side-effects can also be an effective way of tracking what's going on (or proving your point) if you feel like your current contraceptive isn't right for you.

Resources
- Chronic Urinary Tract Infection Campaign – cutic.co.uk
- Decolonising Contraception – decolonisingcontraception.com
- Lichen Sclerosus Awareness – instagram.com/lichens-clerosusuk

- OMGYES – omgyes.com
- Pudendal Neuralgia Awareness – instagram.com/pnawareness_uk_
- Sexwise – sexwise.org.uk
- Sling the Mesh – slingthemeshcampaign.org
- Terrence Higgins Trust – tht.org.uk
- The Lowdown – theldown.com
- The Vaginismus Network – thevaginismusnetwork.com
- Vulval Pain Society – vulvalpainsociety.org

7

'The war on cancer': Gendering the C word

Cancer. The big C. Whatever you call it, it undoubtedly occupies a much bigger place in the public consciousness than many of the issues we've talked about so far – and understandably so. One in two of us will get cancer in our lifetime, and all of us will be touched in some way by its effects. As health issues go it's about as well known and universal as they come and the world's largest independent cancer charity, Cancer Research UK, receives funding of more than £600 million a year, including almost £200 million from donations. Cancer is a disease that we all, patients and clinicians alike, take seriously.

Data from the National Cancer Research Institute (NCRI) shows that breast cancer – the most common cancer in women – consistently receives more research funding in the UK than any other cancer. Breast cancer is one of the 'big four' cancers in terms of death rate, with only lung and bowel cancer accounting for a larger proportion of cancer deaths each year in the UK. However, as the NCRI data shows, the research funding is not applied proportionately.

Lung cancer, which in 2014 accounted for 22% of cancer deaths, received £14.6 million in funding. Bowel (colorectal) cancer, accounting for 10.3% of cancer deaths, received £25 million in funding. But breast cancer, accounting for 7.7% of cancer deaths, received over £40 million, more than both combined. Meanwhile, the fourth biggest cancer in the UK, prostate cancer, accounted for 6.5% of deaths, but received little more than half the funding at £22 million. The latest NCRI data shows not much has changed, with breast cancer still topping the funding charts by some distance in 2019/20.

So, what does cancer have to do with the gender health gap? Surely, when it comes to cancer at least, women are doing pretty well. If only it was that simple. Sadly, breast cancer – and even then only primary breast cancer – is the exception rather than the rule when it comes to funding for female-dominated cancers. While breast cancer research received almost £52 million in 2019/20, rarer cancers like vulval and vaginal cancer, for example, found themselves near the bottom of the heap, with just over £180,000 spent on each. All five gynaecological cancers – womb, cervical, ovarian, vulval and vaginal – combined received around £15 million, with £9 million of that going to ovarian cancer.

'The whole challenge around cancer research is we have these four big cancers, which attract attention, they attract funding, they're easier to talk about and they affect the highest numbers of people. However, 47% of the cancers that people are diagnosed with and 55% of the cancers that people die from are rare cancers – so actually more people die from a rare cancer than one of the big four,' says Athena Lamnisos, CEO of gynaecological cancer charity, the Eve Appeal. The difficulty, she explains, is that researchers focused on any of these rarer cancers are all 'fishing in a much smaller pool' of funding.

With breast cancer in particular, Athena adds, 'There was a huge global research effort drawn together about 20 years ago and they started to see success. Success leads to more research funding, so primary breast cancer has made great strides and everything else has been left behind.' This includes secondary (metastatic or incurable) breast cancer, which tends not to benefit so much from breast cancer research funding, despite being the main cause of breast cancer-related deaths.

'The other challenge is that the lion's share of cancer research funding goes into finding better treatments. With gynae cancers, particularly the really devastating diagnoses like ovarian cancer, it's early diagnosis and prevention that's going to save most lives in the end,' she explains.

Meanwhile, gender and other biases seep into so many aspects of our cultural understanding of cancer. I personally have felt turned off by both the pinkification and the sexualisation of breast cancer fundraising campaigns, for example, although I'm sure that both have played a role in raising the profile of the disease.

Readers of a certain age may remember the mid-2000s Save Kylie's Boobs campaign, a fundraiser for Cancer Research UK set up by a fan following Kylie Minogue's breast cancer diagnosis. As a teenage girl and a baby feminist at the time, I remember feeling queasy about the emphasis on Kylie's sex appeal rather than her health. Was her life not valuable in its own right, with or without her boobs? Was she – and so many other breast cancer patients – somehow worth less following her partial mastectomy? While there's no doubt that celebrity cancer diagnoses give a boost to both fundraising and public awareness, I also couldn't help but wonder if the response would have been different if she'd had bowel cancer or something a bit less... well, sexy.

While I do think both the sexualisation and the broader public messaging around breast cancer have improved since my teens, there's also a broader issue here about palatability and which cancers we feel comfortable talking about. The emergence of brilliant patient-led campaigns like CoppaFeel, for example, have helped shift the breast cancer conversation to self-examination, and knowing the signs and symptoms for early detection and diagnosis. Equally, we are beginning to see similar, vitally important public awareness campaigns around gynaecological cancers, with charities like the Eve Appeal empowering women and those with gynae organs to 'know their normal', confront gynae taboos and get anything unusual checked out. However, the pervasive idea that vulvas and vaginas are 'inappropriate', 'dirty' or 'too sexual' for public discussion is still a barrier to really normalising gynae issues.

'You can imagine being in a hospital or GP setting where they're showing videos about how to check your breasts. Similarly with prostate cancer, I don't think people immediately think of penises or sexualised imagery. One of the potential projects we're reviewing at the moment is to look at how palatable it would be to have something around checking your vulva,' Athena says. 'For us, it's about trying to normalise it and put things on a more equal footing, but how palatable will it be, or will it send everyone shielding their children's eyes? I don't know.'

For all cancers, there's also the use of (often highly gendered) language around 'battling', 'fighting', 'winning' and 'losing' in a 'war against cancer'. As patients of all genders have pointed out, this kind of language is problematic and unhelpful in the way it frames cancer treatment and recovery as a feat of personal strength – an obstacle that can be overcome if only the patient tries hard enough. And, for women in particular, it can often feel as if their bodies, their lives and their wellbeing become collateral damage.

*

The survivorship agenda – which places an emphasis on cancer survivors' long-term health, wellbeing and quality of life, rather than simply keeping them alive at any cost – is one that is increasingly being pushed to the fore by patient advocates. But there are still too many examples of women who have been left feeling that they were unable to give informed consent to painful, traumatic and even life-altering treatments and procedures.

There are, of course, difficult decisions to be made and enormous challenges to be faced with any cancer treatment, whether that's surgery to remove or prevent cancerous tumours, or intensive treatments like chemo and radiotherapy. None of this is easy. Yet I also hear from women and gender minorities about experiences that could have been mitigated – traumatic, invasive and non-consensual incidents during breast and cervical screening; painful LLETZ treatments (large loop excision of the transformation zone, used to remove abnormal cells from the cervix) and hysteroscopy procedures (to examine the inside of the womb); or being wrongly denied the opportunity to preserve their fertility prior to treatment.

Cervical screening is a particularly interesting example and one where I believe we are finally, gradually, starting to see some progress in response to decades of patients voting with their feet and speaking out about their concerns. The UK's cervical screening (or smear test) programme was launched in 1988 and prevents three-quarters of cases of cervical cancer, saving an estimated 5000 lives each year. All women, trans men, non-binary and intersex people with a cervix are eligible for screening. In England and Northern Ireland they're currently invited every three years between the ages of 25 and 49, then every five years until the age of 65, while eligible patients are invited every five years in Scotland and Wales.

However, each year, around a million of those people choose not to attend. By 2018 cervical screening uptake had reached a 21-year low, with one in four of those who were invited opting out. Nine years earlier, reality TV star Jade Goody's death from cervical cancer, aged just 27, was credited with prompting an extra 400,000 women to go for screening, but this 'Jade Goody effect' was short-lived. Meanwhile, previous awareness campaigns have been accused of being too reductive about the reasons for this, or trivialising and dismissing screening hesitancy as just 'embarrassment'. So, what is really going on?

The screening process itself has changed very little from the 'pap smear' developed by Georgios Papanikolaou in the 1940s and uses a speculum, the original design for which was pioneered nearly 200 years ago by James Marion Sims. You might remember him from earlier as the so-called 'Father of Modern Gynaecology', whose medical legacy was built on hugely unethical experiments carried out on Black enslaved women. The design of the speculum, which is inserted into the vagina and allows clinicians to open it up to look inside, has changed very little in the last two centuries, although many are now made from plastic rather than metal, and they come in varying sizes.

During the 1970s, second-wave feminists 'saw the speculum as an instrument of power that physicians used against women', according to researcher Margarete Sandelowski, and objected to the vulnerable positions – naked, on their backs, with a stranger peering into their vagina – that gynaecology required women to take at the hands of (often male) healthcare professionals. Although cervical screening today is typically done by (mostly female) practice nurses, and patients can specifically request a female smear-taker, the vulnerability and unequal power dynamic of the screening process remains a huge barrier for survivors of sexual violence and other traumas, as well as patients living with gender dysphoria, vaginismus, vaginal atrophy or other vulval pain conditions.

It's only really in the last few years that we've begun to see any real acknowledgement of, and work done to address, these challenges. A significant factor in this shift came in 2015 with the opening of My Body Back, a survivor-led clinic that offers cervical screening, STI testing and contraceptive care to female and assigned female at birth (AFAB) non-binary survivors of sexual violence. My Body Back now has clinics in London and Glasgow, and charities like Jo's Cervical Cancer Trust and the Eve Appeal also offer information and advice for survivors of sexual violence, as well as training and resources for clinicians on supporting this vulnerable patient group.

Other barriers to screening include the longstanding, but false, belief that lesbians and bisexual women in same-sex relationships are not at risk from HPV (the virus that causes virtually all cases of cervical cancer), and, of course, shame, cultural stigmas and embarrassment – none of which are trivial issues.

For patients with disabilities, there may also be barriers around accessibility, both in terms of physical access for wheelchair users and the availability of accessible, easy-read information and support for those with learning disabilities or autism. Research by Jo's Cervical Cancer Trust found that nearly two-thirds of the physically disabled women they surveyed had been unable to access cervical screening, while research by the charity Dimensions found just 19% of women with a learning disability or autism had had a recent smear test.

In 2019 I interviewed Fiona Anderson, a wheelchair user with muscular dystrophy, who launched a petition calling on the Department for Health and Social Care to make cervical screening accessible. For the previous five years, since turning 25, Fiona had been trying to book her cervical screening, but was told it wouldn't be possible because her local surgery didn't have the hoist that she would need. Trying to reassure her, Fiona's GP had said, 'Your risk of getting cervical cancer is low because you're a wheelchair user [so] you're sexually inactive.'

As a mother of two young children, who definitely weren't conceived through divine intervention, Fiona was aghast at this assumption. 'Just because I'm in a wheelchair, you cannot assume that I don't have a sex life. But even people who aren't sexually active should still have the right to access screening for their own reassurance and peace of mind,' she said. Her petition quickly gained more than 100,000 signatures and, despite delays during the pandemic, Fiona is now working with the Department of Health and Social Care, as well as local MPs, to try to rectify the issues disabled women face with accessing screening.

While there is still clearly much work to be done, where we are beginning to see changes is in the growing recognition that traditional cervical screening simply does not work for everyone and that these issues run much deeper than just silly little women being embarrassed about their private parts. As a result, we've also seen a flurry of largely women-led innovation to design alternatives. In the US, for example, the all-female team of designers and engineers behind Yona Care have reimagined the speculum, with what they claim is a body-friendly design for a more patient-centred approach to pelvic examinations. Notable features include a 'three-leaved design [to provide] a clear field-of-view without opening the speculum uncomfortably wide', and silicone-covered stainless steel, 'reducing coldness and making insertion less painful'.

Meanwhile, in the UK, researchers led by Dr Emma Crosbie at the University of Manchester and Dr Belinda Nedjai at Queen Mary University of London have seen promising results in trials that used urine samples to screen for high-risk forms of HPV. Similarly, DIY screening kits – which use a self-taken vaginal (rather than cervical) swab to test for high-risk HPV – are now being piloted in the UK, having been successfully used in Australia, Denmark and the Netherlands for years.

The idea behind both these approaches is to provide a non-invasive screening process, which would allow women and people with cervixes to collect their samples themselves in the comfort of their own homes, before sending them off for lab analysis. While there is still an important place for clinician examinations when it comes to gynae health – and we must also find ways of making this more comfortable – it's hoped that the emergence of self-sampling techniques could help to reach those who aren't currently being screened at all.

*

It's worth remembering that cervical cancer is the only cancer with a screening programme designed to prevent cancer from ever developing, as opposed to catching it in the early stages, as with breast and bowel cancer screening. For all other cancers then – as well as some cervical cancers, which screening may miss – early diagnosis and treatment is almost always dependent on patients identifying early signs, their GPs recognising these symptoms, and an appropriate and timely referral being made. Here again, though, we see issues with women's accounts of their symptoms being minimised or disbelieved, which can have serious consequences.

Dafina Malovska and Clare Baumhauer, both of whom I interviewed in 2019, are prime examples. Clare had suffered from a sore, itchy vulva for the best part of 40 years, since primary school, and been repeatedly misdiagnosed, often without so much as an examination. She was sent away with thrush creams, told she had cystitis, eczema and even herpes. 'I must have been seen 30 times over the years, by different doctors, with the same symptoms. Most of them didn't even look at my vulva, I was just told I had a yeast infection,' she told me. In 2016, Clare was diagnosed with vulval cancer – a rare consequence, in her case, of lichen sclerosus.

As I mentioned in chapter 6, this is a chronic inflammatory skin condition. Although there's no cure it can be managed using steroid creams and patients should receive lifetime monitoring, because the condition slightly increases their risk of vulval or penile cancers. This is rare – around 1% of women in the UK are affected by lichen sclerosus and only around 5% of those cases will develop into vulval cancer. However, having never been diagnosed, Clare had never received any treatment or monitoring.

'I've had two babies, I've had smear tests every three years and no nurse or midwife had ever picked up on it,' she said. 'If I'd been diagnosed with lichen sclerosus as a child, been treated and monitored all my life, I might still have got cancer. But I definitely would have gone back to my GP much sooner and the cancer could have been caught earlier.'

As a result of her experiences, Clare now uses social media to raise awareness of the signs and symptoms of both lichen sclerosus and vulval cancer. Similarly, Dafina Malovska launched her Check Me Up campaign, calling for regular women's health checks, after her womb cancer was dismissed as a gluten intolerance. At 35, Dafina was advised to cut out wheat and 'eat Activia yogurts' after experiencing severe and persistent bloating. 'Every time I went back to see my GP, I could tell from her reaction that she thought I was a hypochondriac. She never actually touched my abdomen or examined me, not even once,' she said.

After experiencing bleeding between periods, Dafina was eventually referred to gynaecology, but in the meantime consulted a private gynaecologist in her native Macedonia. Following a transvaginal ultrasound and pelvic examination, they discovered a 14cm, 500g tumour in her uterus – which surgery later revealed was stage two womb cancer. That same evening she underwent a total hysterectomy and oophorectomy, removing both her uterus and ovaries, and putting her into an early surgical menopause.

With no time to process her situation prior to the surgery, the anger and grief at losing her fertility as a single, childless 35-year-old only kicked in afterwards. 'It was very, very difficult. There were some days when I just felt lost,' she told me. 'The tumour was so big by the time they found it and I realised so much of this could have been prevented if someone had examined me earlier.'

Part of the problem, Eve Appeal's Athena Lamnisos believes, is that GPs tend to reach for the most likely or obvious answer, instead of ruling out cancer as their first port of call. This is particularly true with younger patients like Clare and Dafina, among whom cancer is less common. 'GPs have got to know about absolutely everything and unfortunately, when it comes to rare diseases, they are not specialists. Likewise with gynaecological issues, GPs have varying levels of training and expertise,' she says.

That said, all GPs should have enough knowledge of women's health to be able to identify red flags. 'A GP trainee will attend half-day training sessions and spend some of the time during their GP placements dealing with women's health concerns,' explains Dr Anne Connolly MBE, a GP with a special interest in women's health. 'Once qualified as a GP we need to demonstrate ongoing learning in all aspects of primary care, so even GPs who don't specialise in women's health will have to do some training in it at some point,' she adds.

All GPs should therefore be ruling out cancer and other serious conditions, Anne says, before following the pathway of 'common things happen commonly'. Experience, she adds, is the most useful tool for that. 'We also have the advantage of time, so we can set a plan to follow up if the condition continues or worsens, or refer to someone else who may have more experience in the subject matter.'

In practice, however, Athena says: 'The way it often seems to work is that GPs rule out the most common or likely explanations first – such as thrush or digestive issues – so you get this big delay before they consider cancer.' With a symptom like abnormal vaginal bleeding, she explains, in post-menopausal women that would now trigger a two-week referral for cancer investigations, but with younger women there are many other possible causes for abnormal bleeding that are more likely. What you also get, Athena adds, is a sort of dissonance of: 'You're too young', 'You don't fit', because the person in front of them doesn't look like someone who would typically have cancer.

As both Clare and Dafina found, there's also an issue with GPs feeling reluctant to examine patients – and those patients being reluctant to suggest it. 'GPs often don't look and that's partly because there's this preconceived bias all the way through healthcare of GPs thinking that people are embarrassed to be examined, or there's not enough time, or it's too invasive to examine someone,' Athena says.

'It really only involves a question: "Would you be happy for me to examine you?" But with vulval and ovarian cancer we know it can take five or six visits before someone is examined or even just palpated (touched to feel for any issues). If the patient is also not looking themselves, they won't know, for example, what their vulva looks like normally and therefore won't notice if anything's changed. They may also have pain and discomfort that goes on for a long, long time before they actually even go to see the GP,' she adds.

These are all serious challenges for GPs – particularly, as Anne points out, when gynae cancers like ovarian cancer are often quite vague in the way they present. Nevertheless, she adds, much more is needed to address healthcare inequalities and ensure women like Dafina and Clare don't slip through the cracks. For the Eve Appeal, normalising these kinds of conversations between GPs and their patients, and improving awareness of the signs and symptoms of all five gynaecological cancers, are vital steps towards improving the UK's early diagnosis rates and, ultimately, saving more lives. 'Education and empowerment needs to happen from both sides – patient to doctor and doctor to patient,' Athena says. 'Women must feel able to discuss their concerns and find relevant information to understand when they should seek medical help, how to appropriately push for answers if their symptoms persist, and how to agree a joint plan with their doctor.'

There are, though, as we've seen, significant social and cultural barriers to opening up these conversations on both sides – from the fact that British women simply aren't used to intimate examinations in the way that many of our counterparts are in the US and parts of Europe (where regular 'Well Woman' health checks are more common), to the broader stigmas and taboos that still surround our vulvas, vaginas and other gynaecological anatomy. Indeed, while there's evidence that the 3–5 year interval of cervical screening in the UK helps reduce the risk of needless over-treatment, I can also understand the argument that more regular gynae checks (typically only available privately in the UK) might improve our comfort and familiarity with the more intimate parts of our bodies.

∗

For trans men and non-binary people who were assigned female at birth, there are also significant logistical barriers, as well as anti-trans bias from healthcare professionals, that get in the way. Anyone who is born with a uterus, cervix, ovaries, vulva, vagina and breasts, and who hasn't had surgery to remove any combination of those, is at risk of the cancers affecting these body parts.

While most but not all trans men and trans masculine people choose to have 'top surgery' as part of their gender-affirming treatment, many more won't have 'bottom surgery'. Some may choose only the removal of the womb and/or ovaries. However, the way NHS systems currently work means that, if they're registered as male with their GP surgery, they may not automatically be invited for cervical or breast screening and may also have difficulties accessing other forms of gynaecological care.

Ben is trans masculine and tells me about his experience of being investigated for an ovarian cyst. 'They needed to do a set of tests to check if it was cancerous, but the NHS system wouldn't allow them to book these tests as I was in the system as male,' he explains. As a result, Ben adds, his investigations were delayed by several weeks and he had to come back at a later date. Fortunately, when he was eventually referred for testing, it came back all clear, but for someone who says he's a natural worrier with a family history of cancer, the delays were an extra source of stress and anxiety that should have been wholly avoidable.

Many of the trans people I've spoken to are all too aware of the risks associated with anti-trans bias in healthcare, particularly when it comes to life-threatening conditions like cancer. The 2001 documentary film *Southern Comfort* tells the story of American trans man Robert Eades, who was diagnosed with ovarian cancer in 1996. Robert was refused treatment by more than a dozen doctors. By the time he found someone willing to treat him, the cancer had metastasised, spreading to other parts of his body, and was incurable. He died in 1999. While stories like Robert's are rare, the attitudes behind them sadly aren't, even more than two decades later.

When Ben's first cervical screening appointment was due, he had to request an appointment himself. 'As trans people we're essentially told that by having our gender corrected on the GP system they take no responsibility for our care; the systems do not account for our bodies, so it's up to us to know what we need to get monitored and when,' he explains.

It took a lot of psyching himself up even to get Ben to a point where he felt comfortable booking the appointment. But, once there, he was faced with 'very heteronormative assumptions and questions', before being given the same misinformation often handed out to lesbian and bisexual women: that, although he was sexually active in other ways, he didn't need screening because he wasn't having penis-in-vagina sex.

'It was only by accessing trans spaces online that I found people who explained that's not right – anyone with a cervix should be screened. Trans people have to become our own doctors to find this stuff out,' he explains. 'This was really frustrating, but also defeating, because it meant I would have to build myself up to going again.' As a result, at 27, Ben has still not had his first cervical screening test, but is hoping to attend a trans-specific clinic in London to have it done in a more supportive and understanding environment. 'I wouldn't return to a regular service for my smear test; it's only recently that I've finally followed this issue up with a trans-specific clinic,' he adds.

Jack, who shared his experiences of trans broken arm syndrome earlier, also encountered difficulties with cervical screening. 'I found my cervical smear test quite painful because of vaginal atrophy [thinning and dryness, caused by testosterone treatment]. The nurse just laughed at me and said, "You're a man now, you should be able to deal with pain." That again is very standard, and such a horrible and toxic stereotype. You shouldn't be telling anyone that,' he says.

This kind of unsympathetic approach from healthcare professionals – in Jack's case also steeped in toxic stereotypes about masculinity – is not uncommon, as surveys on trans people's healthcare experiences frequently show. Dr Alison Berner is a medical oncologist and gender specialist, whose research has looked at trans men and non-binary people's attitudes to cervical screening. 'Anticipated stigma or discrimination is a big barrier to trans people attending cervical screening, either because it's happened to other people they have heard about or they themselves have had bad interactions,' she explains. 'We've also seen cases of healthcare professionals being a bit over familiar – where they're trying to be supportive but getting it wrong, like commenting on changes to their body or saying how well they pass for cisgender now, and then the patient just wants to get the hell out of the room.'

Alison believes sensitive, trans-inclusive care should be embedded as part of basic communication skills throughout medical school curricula. 'You need to know to ask the right questions and build trust. It's about understanding what to say and what not to say, and how to be led by the patient. All of that starts with friendly, open and sensitive communication, even before any of the medical stuff,' she says. 'I think today's undergraduates are much more accepting than previous generations, but there are still underlying stigmas and discrimination, as well as those (generally more established) doctors who are broadly accepting of trans patients but just not willing to learn.'

Meanwhile, on a more practical level, she adds, the NHS needs a cervical screening system that works for all patients, not just most of them, both in terms of the information provided and the IT systems used to send out screening invitations. A more inclusive system, based on anatomy rather than gender, has been mooted in recent years, but is yet to materialise. Instead, by relying solely on a patient's gender marker, the current system not only sees trans men being excluded and trans women being erroneously invited, but also results in screening invitations being sent to cis women who no longer have a cervix, including those who've had it removed as part of previous cancer treatment. The implications of this will range from mildly irritating to traumatic for those women who are invited in error, and potentially life-threatening for trans men and others who are excluded. Although planned changes should make it easier for patients to opt in and out, the onus is still on trans patients to know what healthcare they need and to proactively seek it out.

It might therefore seem surprising that some of the most vicious parts of the 'gender wars' in recent years have attacked efforts to make cancer prevention and early diagnosis more inclusive of trans people. The use of inclusive language, like 'cis women, trans men, non-binary and intersex people with a cervix', is admittedly a bit of a mouthful when talking about those at risk of certain cancers, but it's also the most accurate and inclusive way of ensuring everyone is aware of the risks relevant to their anatomy. Yet gynae cancer charities and health advocates alike have been met with fury and accusations of 'erasing women' for daring to allow for such nuance in their information. Meanwhile, even politicians – many of them clueless and poorly briefed – have waded into distracting and harmful arguments about who does or doesn't have a cervix.

Much less ire, interestingly, has been heaped on charities, including Macmillan Cancer Support and Prostate Cancer UK, who use language like 'men, trans women and people assigned male at birth' to accurately describe who is at risk of prostate cancer. The simple reality, though, is that everyone, regardless of their gender or trans status, deserves equal access to information and services that could prevent, diagnose and treat cancer – particularly as we know transition itself can reduce the risk of some cancers, while increasing the risk of others.

Trans women, for example, are 48 times more at risk of breast cancer than cis men, but three times less at risk than cis women. They're still at risk of prostate cancer, but testosterone-blocking treatment makes their risk lower than in cis men. However, for trans women who have not had lower surgery, the use of hormonal therapy does not appear to reduce the risk of testicular cancer. Given these varying risks, doctors do need to be aware of their trans patients' anatomy and treatment history, rather than simply treating them as exactly the same as either cis men or cis women.

This is true across healthcare, Alison says, and is not helped by the limited amount of available research into trans patients' health and relative risks. 'Not being able to disaggregate sex and gender in healthcare data means we don't necessarily know what advice to give trans people, which can often end up with suboptimal results. In a lot of cases we don't know whether it's hormones, behaviour or chromosomes that determine the risk. Understanding that better will actually help us treat everybody better, whether they're trans or cisgender,' Alison says.

✳

Gendered issues with cancer care can also be seen in some of the diagnostic and preventative procedures used, like LLETZ and hysteroscopy – although, to be clear, these treatments can be lifesaving. LLETZ, which stands for 'large loop excision of the transformation zone', is used to remove pre-cancerous cervical cell changes which, if left untreated, could develop into cervical cancer. Meanwhile, hysteroscopy is an endoscopic procedure used to detect womb cancer, among other uterine issues. Yet thousands of women have reported that they weren't properly informed about potential pain and after-effects associated with the procedures.

Jocelyn Lewis is a member of the Campaign Against Painful Hysteroscopy (CAPH), founded in 2014 by patient-led advocacy group Hysteroscopy Action. Jocelyn was referred for a scan and exploratory hysteroscopy in 2017, under the two-week urgent cancer referral scheme, after experiencing post-menopausal bleeding – a potential red flag for womb cancer. Writing for Hysterical Women two years later, she describes the experience as 'the most painful moment of my life'.

Hysteroscopy involves passing a narrow telescopic camera into the womb, through the vagina and cervix, to investigate, diagnose and in some cases treat problems like unexplained or abnormal vaginal bleeding or pelvic pain. In many respects it's similar to a colonoscopy, which is used to investigate bowel issues. However, as Hysteroscopy Action highlights, patients who undergo an NHS colonoscopy are routinely offered a choice of pain relief in the form of Entonox (gas and air) or IV sedation with analgesia. For the women and patients with wombs undergoing hysteroscopy, however, the standard advice is to take a couple of paracetamol or ibuprofen beforehand. 'Are women assumed to have higher pain thresholds? Or are we just expected to put up and shut up?' Jocelyn asks.

While over-the-counter painkillers are enough for many women to manage the mild pain and discomfort they experience, NHS England pain audits obtained by Hysteroscopy Action show that around one in four hysteroscopy outpatients experience severe pain, rated as 7/10 or more. This is particularly the case for post-menopausal women and those who haven't given birth but, as with the pain associated with IUD insertion, it can be difficult to predict who will or won't be badly affected.

When Jocelyn went in for her hysteroscopy, she'd already read some disturbing stories online and mentioned to her consultant that she was worried it would be painful. 'He repeatedly dismissed all my concerns and said, "No, not at all, at worst something akin to light period pain,"' she says. 'As women and mothers we go through many medical examinations which are unpleasant, and during which we feel extremely exposed and vulnerable. I was, however, in no way prepared for the horrendous pain of hysteroscopy,' Jocelyn adds, describing the experience of having the metal hysterosope forced through her cervix as 'barbaric'.

'I was crying; I couldn't speak; I could feel myself passing out. Two nurses, who didn't seem surprised at my reaction, were either side of me, trying to calm me down. I now know this is the NHS' cheap alternative to anaesthetic – 'vocal local' – designed for use in Third World countries as a distraction technique. The horror continued as fluid was pumped into my womb,' she continues.

It was only towards the end of the procedure that the consultant offered to stop, adding that Jocelyn would have to come back and have the procedure done again. 'There was no suggestion that I could come back and have it done under anaesthetic or conscious sedation. I was in no state to be able to discuss anything rationally. I was barely conscious,' Jocelyn explains. 'I was there to see if I had cancer and that was all I could focus on, so I felt I had no choice but to allow him to complete the procedure.'

Fortunately, doctors found no sign of cancer – something Jocelyn says she will always be extremely grateful for. However, her hysteroscopy experience had a profound effect on her and prompted her to begin campaigning with CAPH. The campaign's main aims are for full written information about the procedure to be provided, including the honest risk of severe pain, and for safe and effective pain relief to be offered as standard – with patients given a genuine choice between no anaesthetic, local anaesthesia, safely monitored conscious sedation, epidural or general anaesthesia. Here too there are already promising moves in the right direction. The RCOG (Royal College of Obstetricians and Gynaecologists) is due to publish a good practice paper on pain relief and informed decision making for outpatient hysteroscopy procedures in early 2023. This is expected to recommend that all pain relief options should be discussed with patients, as well as the risks and benefits of each. This, Jocelyn points out, would enable all patients to make a fully informed choice – and give fully informed consent – about their care.

Similarly, writer Kate Orson launched the Intact Cervix campaign after experiencing unexpected side-effects following the LLETZ procedure. Writing for Hysterical Women in 2018, she said: 'Hundreds of women, myself included, have found ourselves experiencing side-effects that our doctors never warned us about. We have found that we've lost sexual function, that our libido plummets, that our orgasms become weaker and that sex becomes painful. Women are finding they experience vaginal dryness, problems with constipation, incontinence and

THE WAR ON CANCER

pelvic pain. There are other "whole body" effects too, such as nausea, fatigue and headaches.'

Through a Facebook support group, she added: 'We've found that one thing is common to almost all of us: that doctors deny and minimise our side-effects. They tell us that they are "all in our heads" and aren't related to the LLETZ. Women have been told to seek counselling rather than being given adequate medical treatment for the problems they are facing.' This dismissiveness, Kate believes, is at least in part down to the fact that most doctors have little to no knowledge of the role of the cervix in sexual function and orgasm. When you combine this with the fact that, as we saw in chapter 6, women's sexual pleasure is rarely prioritised, it's easy to see why these side-effects have so often and so easily been brushed aside.

But the impact on women's emotional, romantic and sexual lives is real and profound. According to a 2019 survey on patient experiences of LLETZ and other treatments for cervical cell changes, published by Jo's Cervical Cancer Trust, 33% of respondents had experienced pain during or after sex, with 25% of those experiencing symptoms for more than five years after treatment. The survey also found that 22% had experienced bleeding during or after sex, and 46% had experienced psychological changes impacting on their relationships and sex lives. Among the women Kate has heard from, some have separated from their partners and some even live with PTSD.

Not only are these side-effects not well enough known about and women not well enough informed, but Kate believes there's a sexist double standard in the way men's and women's sexual functions are prioritised in cancer treatment and prevention. One clinical trial in Germany, she points out, saw men with prostate cancer given advanced robotic surgery that aimed 'to preserve the fine architecture of microscopic nerves around the prostate – and with them the patient's sexual function.'

The report from Jo's Cervical Cancer Trust is clear that more research is needed to properly understand the after-effects reported by women like Kate, improve the consistency of information offered to patients, and properly recognise the impact that a diagnosis of cervical cell changes and associated treatments can have. Besides the lesser-known sexual side-effects highlighted by Kate's campaign, more common side-effects of LLETZ and similar treatments include bleeding, spotting or pain for up to four weeks afterwards, changes to vaginal discharge, and infection. More rarely, scarring of the cervical opening (known as cervical stenosis) can occur, causing a partial or full blockage of the passage between the womb and the vagina. There's also around a 2% risk of premature birth among people who become pregnant at any time after the LLETZ procedure.

There's an issue here around over-treatment as well. There are three different grades of cervical changes. CIN1 is classed as low grade and not requiring treatment, while CIN3 is high grade and treatment is always offered. However, also in 2019, Jo's Trust reported inconsistencies with how the middle ground, CIN2, is managed – with some patients offered treatment straight away, while others were monitored to keep an eye on changes.

Given the severity of side-effects that some women experience after LLETZ, this more conservative approach certainly seems preferable and the latest evidence supports that. A review published by the *BMJ* in 2018 concluded that most CIN2 changes, particularly in younger women, get better by themselves and can therefore be managed through 'active surveillance' every six months to check for any changes to the cells. For many years, though, this decision has been left to the discretion of individual clinicians. Updated guidance on this was due to be published by the British Society for Colposcopy and Cervical Pathology, but so far nothing has changed.

For women who are offered this procedure, clearly there is a difficult decision to be made. As Kate says: 'When faced with a choice between an invasive procedure that may destroy your sex life, or the chance of developing cancer, many women would opt for the treatment.' But, she adds, 'the fact is that women haven't been given this informed choice. Abnormalities are not cancer and no illness gives doctors the licence to bypass their legal obligation to informed consent.'

Indeed, while just 4% of the patients surveyed by Jo's said they wished they had not received treatment, many more reported they felt ill-informed and 20% said they were not warned about any possible side-effects. Equally, Kate says: 'If women do decide the LLETZ is the best option, they need proper support afterwards and acknowledgement of what has happened.' The way she and others have seen doctors respond instead – whether a result of ignorance or gaslighting – only adds to their trauma.

∗

Infertility is another of the possible side-effects of cancer treatment that we tend not to think or talk so much about. But, particularly for young cancer patients, the issue of their fertility can be one of the most pressing concerns. Depending on the type and location of the cancer, treatments like chemotherapy and radiotherapy – as well as any surgery on reproductive anatomy – can cause later fertility problems or infertility. Guidelines state that 'the impact of cancer and its treatment on future fertility' should be discussed with all cancer patients at diagnosis and that cryopreservation – freezing of eggs, sperm or embryos – should be offered. However, particularly for women, this option isn't always forthcoming.

I first met Becki McGuinness in early 2017, shortly after she'd launched her Cancer and Fertility UK campaign, and seven years after she lost her own fertility through a combination of chemo and radiotherapy. Becki had been diagnosed with osteosarcoma – a rare and aggressive form of bone cancer – when she was just 21 years old. With the cancer located in her sacrum and lower spine, Becki was told radiotherapy targeting the area around her pelvis could have an impact on her fertility. Despite this, Becki told me, her concerns were brushed off by the doctors in her cancer team, who insisted there was no time and no other options, but reassured her that infertility 'doesn't happen to everyone.'

After taking her doctors at their word, Becki was devastated when pelvic radiotherapy put her into an early menopause, leaving her infertile. The ultimate kick in the teeth came later, though, when a fertility specialist told her there would have been enough time to preserve her fertility prior to starting treatment. 'If the oncologists had told me there was enough time, even if I'd had to go private, I would have found a way. But that choice was taken away from me,' she said.

'For me, it's a pro-choice issue. If you want to try to preserve your fertility first then, as long as there's time, that choice should be there. It just doesn't feel like they see the whole person, what you will lose and how it will affect you,' Becki adds. Yet, the more she researched it, the more she realised her own experience was not an isolated incident: 'It was happening to lots of women.'

In fact, research published in 2017 found that less than 4% of female cancer patients were having their eggs or embryos frozen before undergoing cancer treatment. The study by St Mary's Hospital Manchester found that around half of female cancer patients aged 15 to 39 – around 4000 a year – are left infertile after their treatment. However, in 2014, just 154 of those women had cryopreservation funded by the NHS. Researchers found a postcode lottery in funding for this service, with as many as two-thirds of women having to pay privately for IVF treatment.

Speaking to the *Daily Mail* at the time, researcher Dr Cheryl Fitzgerald, a consultant in reproductive medicine at St Mary's, said: 'There is a huge inequity. Men having fertility-damaging treatment are automatically referred to sperm banking. For women, because egg freezing used to be less successful and because it's a more invasive and time-consuming process, it's not automatic. The emphasis has obviously been on curing cancer, but with so many people surviving cancer, we need to look at improving the quality of life after treatment, including the chance to have a family.'

YOUR CANCER TOOLKIT

When it comes to cancer, knowledge really is power, as early diagnosis and intervention can make all the difference. Get to know your body, identify which cancers are relevant to your anatomy and tune in to what's 'normal' for you, so that you can quickly identify if anything changes. This doesn't just mean checking your breasts every month as campaigns like Coppafeel have drummed into us, but also knowing (if applicable to you) your menstrual cycle, and what your vulva and vagina look and feel like.

The symptoms of different cancers are many and various, but as a general rule you should get anything that's unusual for you checked out by your GP, including, but definitely not limited to: bleeding between periods, after sex, or after the menopause; changes to vaginal discharge; persistent bloating; any lumps, bumps, sores, skin changes, new or changed moles; persistent pain or itching; unexplained changes in bowel or bladder habits; and difficulty eating and feeling full quickly.

It might feel melodramatic, but if you're concerned about a potential cancer symptom, don't be afraid to ask your doctor to rule that out first to put your mind at ease. It might be that they can do so immediately, in which case ask them to justify *why* they don't think it's cancer, or it may prompt them to investigate further if it's not something they'd already considered. If they don't offer to examine you, and you feel safe and comfortable doing so, ask them to have a look or a feel.

For symptoms of any of the five gynaecological cancers – womb, cervical, ovarian, vulval and vaginal – the Eve Appeal has a great selection of tips on their website about how to 'talk gynae' with your GP. These include knowing your cycle, using the correct anatomical terminology, and coming prepared with a timeline of your symptoms.

Likewise, if you find cervical screening difficult for any reason, both they and Jo's Trust have tips on coping with the process, including advice specific to survivors of sexual violence and trans/non-binary patients. A double appointment may be helpful, allowing you to take the screening process at your own pace, and remember that you can ask for a smaller speculum to be used, or to insert it yourself.

When it comes to other procedures and treatments, remember you have the right to give fully informed consent, based on the best information available. Do your research and ask about risks, benefits and alternatives when faced with any decision about your care. Although keeping you alive should be everyone's number one priority, you don't have to immediately accept every option that's presented to you; you are allowed to ask for more time, more information or a second opinion, and to say 'no' or 'stop' if you're uncomfortable at any point.

Resources
- Breast Cancer Now – breastcancernow.org
- Campaign Against Painful Hysteroscopy – hysteroscopyaction.org.uk
- Cancer and Fertility UK – cancerandfertility.co.uk
- Coppafeel – coppafeel.org
- Eve Appeal – eveappeal.org.uk
- Intact Cervix – intactcervix.com
- Jo's Cervical Cancer Trust – jostrust.org.uk
- Live Through This – LGBTQ+ cancer support – livethroughthis.co.uk
- Ovacome – ovacome.org.uk
- Ovarian Cancer Action – ovarian.org.uk
- Peaches Womb Cancer Trust – peachestrust.org
- Prostate Cancer UK – prostatecanceruk.org
- Target Ovarian Cancer – targetovariancancer.org.uk
- Trekstock – young adult cancer support – trekstock.com

8

'Baby blues': Perinatal care and the price of motherhood

Earlier I mentioned Gloria Steinem's 'If Men Could Menstruate' essay and I often wonder what the pregnancy and childbirth equivalent would look like. For all the joy and wonder, bringing new life into the world also comes with a whole new layer of gendered baggage – not least when it comes to healthcare.

Rebecca Schiller, who founded the perinatal human rights charity Birthrights, reflects on her time as a doula in her book *Why Human Rights in Childbirth Matter*: 'In birth rooms I witnessed things that I could barely believe could happen in contemporary England. The tendrils of a patriarchy I'd never realised had much to do with me were so firmly entangled in maternity care.'

Feminism has long critiqued the idea of women as 'vessels' or 'incubators' when fighting for access to contraception and abortion. But what about those women who are carrying planned, wanted pregnancies? How often do their identities dissolve into 'Mum' from the moment they first check in with their midwife? How soon do the feelings and needs of this nameless 'mum' slide down the priority list, eclipsed by the needs of her unborn child?

At Hysterical Women, and in my wider work, I've heard horrifying stories of expectant and labouring mothers being dismissed, both with physical signs that something is wrong in their bodies and with distressing perinatal mental health problems. Besides the natural risks of injury or complications associated with childbirth, there are issues around informed consent, obstetric violence and birthing people being coerced, dismissed or ignored – all of which contribute to the estimated 30,000 traumatic births each year in the UK.

In 1995, Clare Norton gave birth to her second daughter, Lara Sian Crofts, by induction. Clare's eldest, Amy, had also been induced, so she had a pretty good idea of what to expect. 'When I went in to be induced, a student midwife thought the baby was breech, but a senior midwife dismissed this and told the student off for mentioning it in front of me,' she recalls. However, from the start of the induction, Clare knew something was wrong. She describes the pain as constant – a continuous, never-ending contraction – but the midwife insisted she wasn't in labour, told her not to be a baby and turned the drip up. After that, Clare says she doesn't remember much more than a blur of horrendous pain. Lara was born breech and not breathing just an hour after the midwife had told Clare she wasn't in labour. She later died at just eight days old.

More than 25 years after Lara's death, how much has really changed? It's no secret that there are significant safety concerns about NHS maternity units, with 38% of them, at the time of writing, rated as 'requires improvement' by the Care Quality Commission (CQC). In October 2020, the CQC announced plans to target poorly performing maternity units, following high-profile scandals at Shrewsbury and Telford Hospital Trust and East Kent Hospitals Trust.

The Ockenden Review into failings at Shrewsbury and Telford, led by maternity expert Donna Ockenden, was published in March 2022, concluding that maternity staff had not listened to mothers, blamed them for the deaths of their babies, and failed to treat them with kindness and compassion. It also highlighted a culture in which 'natural' birth was prioritised seemingly at any cost, with babies dying after their mothers had been refused Caesarean deliveries. 'The reasons for these failures are clear,' Ockenden said. 'There were not enough staff, there was a lack of ongoing training, there was a lack of effective investigation and governance at the trust and a culture of not listening to the families involved.'

On top of that, horrifying data from a UK programme called Mothers and Babies: Reducing Risk through Audits and Confidential Enquiries (MBRRACE), which monitors and investigates maternal and infant deaths, highlights that racial bias makes Black mothers four times more likely than their white counterparts to die during pregnancy and labour, while Asian mothers are twice as likely to die.

Women have been giving birth since the dawn of humanity and there's no doubt that medical care has come a long way. Yet it's hard not to think that a lot more resources might have been invested in substantially improving the whole experience by now if it involved pushing something the size of a watermelon out of any part of the male anatomy. Instead, we come back to the idea that pain, trauma and suffering are an inevitable part of being a woman.

*

Take hyperemesis gravidarum (HG), the extreme form of morning sickness made briefly famous by Catherine, Princess of Wales, who suffered with it during her pregnancies. While 70–80% of pregnant people experience some nausea and vomiting, HG affects an estimated 1% of those. The condition can be utterly debilitating – so much so that 5% of women with HG end up terminating their pregnancies and more than 50% of them consider it.

Charlotte Howden suffered with HG while pregnant with her son in 2015. Her sickness was so extreme that it left her feeling suicidal and unable to work, yet her GP dismissed it as 'just bad morning sickness'. At 12 weeks pregnant she was admitted to hospital with severe dehydration, and asked doctors to terminate the pregnancy that she and her husband had spent 18 months trying to conceive. Although Charlotte did then receive the treatment she desperately needed, and gave birth in 2016, the experience haunted her throughout the remainder of her pregnancy and beyond.

Like many HG sufferers, Charlotte went on to suffer from postnatal depression. Research suggests women affected by HG are eight times more likely to suffer with anxiety or depression during pregnancy and four times more likely to suffer with postnatal depression. After eventually being diagnosed with PTSD, Charlotte channelled her trauma into activism, creating an online community of HG sufferers and teaming up with producer Lorne Guy to create *Sick – The Battle Against HG*, a 30-minute documentary film on the condition. *Sick*, which premiered on Amazon Prime Video in September 2020, is the first ever documentary on HG and highlights not only the extent to which women suffer with the condition, but also the extent to which they are ignored and dismissed by their doctors.

'There's a continuous thread with every woman I've ever spoken to of their health simply not being considered as important as the health of their baby,' Charlotte says. 'The other common theme is complete miseducation about medication – that if you take this, your baby will be harmed. Everything is concerned about the baby, without looking at what is happening to the woman and the risk-benefit analysis of that.' The irony, she adds, is that, 'By purely looking out for the baby, you inadvertently end up leaving women in such desperation that a termination or suicide feel like the only options.'

Part of Charlotte's campaigning on the subject has been to put pressure on the Royal College of GPs (RCGP) to improve guidance for GPs. However, she also believes healthcare professionals themselves should take more responsibility for improving care. 'Doctors and nurses are totally misinformed about hyperemesis [gravidarum], but equally, if there's a woman in front of you suffering and you don't know why, you bloody well go and find out,' she says.

*

The treatment of women with HG is one of several themes to emerge from the WRISK project, a research collaboration carried out between the British Pregnancy Advisory Service and the School of Social Sciences at Cardiff University to better understand and improve the communication of public health messages around risks in pregnancy. WRISK's principal investigator was Clare Murphy, now chief executive at the British Pregnancy Advisory Service (BPAS).

'While most women obviously want the best for their pregnancies, the focus on the foetus is sometimes at the expense of maternal autonomy and health,' she explains. 'Women accept the precautionary principle that underpins the way we talk about health in pregnancy, but there was a general feeling that access to supporting evidence was not forthcoming.'

This was particularly true, Clare adds, on the issue of medication: 'There was a real point of tension around the acceptance that women have health needs as well. We saw that with women being very sick in pregnancy and also with women who were taking medication for epilepsy or mental health problems.'

In reality, according to consultant obstetric physician Professor Catherine Nelson-Piercy, there is now good evidence to support the use of many drugs during pregnancy, with little to no risk to the foetus. But tragedies like the thalidomide scandal – described as 'the biggest man-made medical disaster ever' – and subsequently the sodium valproate scandal, have made many doctors more cautious about prescribing. Thalidomide, originally prescribed as an anti-sickness medication, caused more than 10,000 children to be born with 'severe and debilitating malformations' during the late 1950s and early 1960s, as well as increased miscarriage rates. Epilepsy drug sodium valproate can also cause birth defects and developmental problems, yet for decades many women on the drug were not warned about these risks. Addressing the latter scandal in her 2020 *First Do No Harm* report, Baroness Julia Cumberlege writes that, by not being given adequate information, 'women were deprived of the ability to make informed decisions about their treatment and family planning options.'

Thousands of women and families were let down by these failings. However, the longer-term impact of both scandals has been an increased anxiety about prescribing any medication at all during pregnancy. In many cases, Clare adds, this leads to women being denied or taken off medication even when there is clear evidence of its safety. 'Women receive the message that these drugs are dangerous to their babies, but they actually put their own health at risk by coming off medicines they need,' Clare says. 'We almost see women's health and foetal health as mutually exclusive, but they go hand in hand.'

In the case of HG, it seems obvious that not being able to keep food and water down poses a risk of malnutrition to the unborn baby, as well as the mother. So why do some doctors focus so heavily on the minimal risks of prescribing anti-sickness medication? While the legacy of thalidomide clearly does cast a long shadow, there's also a sexist and patronising view that pregnancy sickness is 'normal' and a sign of a healthy pregnancy. 'All these roads lead back to the idea that women aren't trusted to accurately report and self-assess; that women just make a fuss,' Clare says.

Another heart-breaking finding from the WRISK research was the dehumanising way in which pregnant women with high BMIs are treated. Many told WRISK researchers they felt like 'a number on a scale', a 'danger whale' and 'a big risk to my baby' – to such an extent that some didn't even put up a cot, because they expected to leave hospital without a baby. In reality, although women with a higher BMI are twice as likely to have a stillbirth, that risk is still very low.

Lack of trust is a clear theme running through antenatal and maternity care, even for pregnant people without underlying health issues, high BMIs or debilitating pregnancy symptoms. 'The message of total abstinence from alcohol in pregnancy is not evidence-based,' Clare says. 'Most women don't want to drink during pregnancy, but you don't need to actively mislead them about the evidence. It's like you can't trust women to understand the difference between an occasional glass of wine and drinking a bottle of wine every night.'

Even more strikingly, Clare adds, 'The greatest manifestation of not trusting women in pregnancy is the carbon monoxide test, which is now routinely carried out during antenatal appointments. A midwife will ask the woman if she smokes and, no matter what her answer, she's given a carbon monoxide test to make sure. Your word is not good enough.'

*

This kind of guilt and blame becomes all the more loaded in the context of pregnancy loss. A close friend suffered a miscarriage while I was writing this chapter. In the midst of her grief, she told me she'd wondered if the loss was her own fault, because the midwife at her booking appointment had made such a fuss about her 'obese' BMI.

An estimated one in four pregnancies end in miscarriage and research published in the *Lancet* medical journal by charity Tommy's in 2021 revealed the devastating mental health impact it can have, doubling both bereaved parents' risk of depression and quadrupling their risk of suicide. Previous research also shows one in five mothers and one in 12 partners experience symptoms of PTSD after miscarriage.

Despite this, many women report not receiving adequate emotional support following pregnancy loss, including during subsequent pregnancies. Lizzie (not her real name), who wrote for Hysterical Women about her experience, described being made to feel like an inconvenience after losing her first pregnancy at nearly 18 weeks. In her second, healthy, pregnancy Lizzie understandably struggled with grief and anxiety – a loss of the innocent excitement and expectation she'd felt the first time around. Yet doctors chastised her for being two pounds overweight and, when she requested a C-section because of her previous trauma, told her: 'Just push it out like millions of other women do.'

Professor Siobhan Quenby is co-author of Tommy's *Lancet* report and deputy director of Tommy's National Centre for Miscarriage Research. According to her: 'Many women have concerns over the unsympathetic care they receive following a miscarriage – with some not being offered any explanation and the only advice they receive being to try again. This is not good enough and we must ensure women are properly supported.'

Hysterical Women contributor Brenda Gabriel wrote of her miscarriage that, 'I have never felt so alone as I did at that moment.' After suffering bleeding during a family trip to Brighton, she was taken to A&E in an ambulance and left to miscarry in a triage room, before being discharged with nothing more than a single information leaflet.

But why does this happen? It's a question without an easy answer, although Siobhan's colleague, Professor Arri Coomarasamy, pondered on it in a blog post for the Royal College of Obstetricians and Gynaecologists (RCOG): 'Is it because it is so common? Is it because people think it wasn't "really a baby", because there weren't any outward signs of a pregnancy? Is it because miscarriage can be seen to be an isolated physical event? Is it because we feel hopeless that nothing can be done to stop a miscarriage?' These misconceptions, he adds, need to be dispelled. Even an early miscarriage is still a profound loss for the person or couple experiencing it and there are concrete steps that can be taken to improve outcomes.

The Tommy's report recommends nationally recording data on miscarriages, as well as establishing clear care pathways for mental health support during and after every loss, and standardised testing and treatments for recurrent miscarriage. In particular, it says, at-risk groups like Black women, women with existing medical conditions and those over 40 should receive care that's personalised to their individual risk factors.

For Brenda, the distress of feeling so abandoned while losing her baby was compounded by an uneasy feeling that the paramedics who attended her at her hotel room were more interested in the dynamic of her mixed-race family than her health. One paramedic, glancing from Brenda to her white partner and their fair-skinned children, asked: 'Are those kids yours?' and she remembers wondering what he was insinuating: 'As a Black woman, did I not fit the picture?'

Although she didn't experience explicit racism during her miscarriage, Brenda's experience is indicative of the implicit biases many women of colour face when accessing healthcare services, perinatal or otherwise. When it comes to miscarriage though, Black women also have a 43% higher risk than white women. This may be linked to their increased risk of type 2 diabetes, heart disease and other health issues, but more research is needed to fully understand the disparity. Combine that with the racial inequalities in maternal mortality, and pregnancy can understandably be a very isolating and anxious time for Black women.

Vanessa Haye has struggled with infertility, IVF treatment, miscarriage and a near-fatal ectopic pregnancy, as well as giving birth to her two sons. Many of these experiences have been riddled with 'misogynoir', as she writes on Hysterical Women. 'It made me realise how the intersection of being both Black and a woman compounds my likelihood of medical gaslighting and adverse treatment outcomes. It felt like I was expected to bear the pain; as if I had an innate and superhuman ability because of the colour and supposed 'thickness' of my skin,' she says.

Vanessa's experiences inspired her to launch online community Femelanin and she's been struck by how pervasive these experiences are among Black women. In campaigning for reproductive justice, she says, it's vital that our activism is rooted in intersectionality. 'At a time when the resurgence of Black Lives Matter has put Black lives at the forefront, we must remember to include the lives of Black women like me.'

*

Many of the same issues crop up during labour. Rebecca Schiller describes the language of childbirth as 'minimising, infantilising and dismissive' – citing examples like 'good girl', 'lack of maternal effort' and 'failure to progress'. Terms like these and 'geriatric mother' were among those targeted by a 2021 'renaming revolution' by Peanut, the social networking app for mothers, which worked with linguists and medical experts to develop a glossary of alternative terms.

Peanut founder Michelle Kennedy describes this language as degrading and rooted in misogyny. But, of course, the roots of that misogyny also go much deeper than words. 'I'm fed up,' Rebecca writes, 'of the dismissal of women's experiences, knowledge, pain and decisions at a time in their lives when supportive care is proven to improve experiences, and when suicide remains the leading indirect cause of maternal death.'

By most standards, giving birth in the UK is safe – just 0.0086% of women will die in childbirth. Yet an estimated one in three women experience some form of traumatic birth, and fear of birth is at an all-time high, so clearly something is going wrong somewhere.

'The dominant cultural narrative is that giving birth is inevitably undignified and intrinsically traumatic. Women and birthing people are discouraged – and often disparaged – for believing that anything more positive is possible. We are often told that nothing matters more than birthing a "healthy baby" when we advocate for our own needs, as if our physical and mental safety, wellbeing and preferences are in competition with those of our foetus. Research and lived experience have repeatedly demonstrated that this presumed conflict is based on deeply flawed assumptions,' Rebecca tells me.

'Dignified, respectful maternity care that prioritises women and birthing people's autonomy, and puts us at the centre of our births, can significantly improve our own physical and mental health outcomes as well as those of our babies – even in more complex pregnancies and births, and especially in groups at greatest risk of a poor outcome. The negative impact of this cultural and clinical gaslighting can be profound, long-lasting and impact significantly on how people experience the start of their parenting journey,' she adds.

Even deeply personal choices about how to give birth aren't always respected. Research published by Birthrights in 2018 revealed the majority of NHS Trusts in the UK make the process of requesting a Caesarean 'lengthy, difficult or inconsistent, adding anxiety and distress to women at a vulnerable time.' In a 2020 survey, carried out by Birthrights and parenting website Mumsnet, one in four women said their wishes about how to give birth were not respected and 14% said their decisions were overruled. What should happen instead, as Rebecca writes in *Why Human Rights in Childbirth Matter*, is for healthcare professionals to 'give women the evidence and trust them to make their own choices.'

Disabled mother Nicola Pennicott-Hall describes her encounter with 'the keeper of the Caesareans' as humiliating and terrifying. Having suffered a spinal injury in her late teens, midwives, obstetricians and anaesthetists all agreed that a planned C-section was the best course of action for Nicola's birth. But the consultant responsible for signing off on the procedure objected, berating Nicola for being 'selfish' and saying she 'couldn't see why' a Caesarean was necessary.

'I was tearful and terrified I was going to be forced to give birth vaginally when I knew I wasn't physically or mentally capable – all because one doctor didn't believe me,' she writes. 'After a heart-stopping few minutes, the consultant capitulated, because she supposed it was "too late to change it," but I was made fully aware of her opinion on the matter.'

There are also serious issues – even in the UK – around obstetric violence. Researcher and childbirth activist Beverley Beech, author of *Am I Allowed?*, describes this as, 'Usually [taking] the form of paternalistic coercion rather than physical violence, ranging from bullying women into agreeing to a range of unnecessary or avoidable interventions, surprisingly often backed up by references to threats of a dead baby or reports to social services if the women do not comply. Most often it consists of disallowing women legitimate decision-making on the grounds that health professionals always know best.'

I remember recently being stopped in my tracks by a post on Instagram account @TheySaidToMe, which documents truly horrifying comments made to pregnant and labouring people by maternity staff, about a woman who had been cut during labour without either her knowledge or consent.

Clearly there's a huge amount to unpick when it comes to women's childbirth experiences, easily enough to fill a separate book (as Rebecca already has), but interviews and guest posts on Hysterical Women reflect the concerns she raises. Time and time again I hear from women who – before, during and after birth – felt they were not heard, believed or taken seriously or that their autonomy and choices were not respected.

Keshet Buckle-Hodgson writes that midwives refused to believe she was in labour during the birth of her first child. 'I was left on a ward, given a ball to sit on, but no medication for pain. I laboured in front of other couples, men and women. Only when I began vomiting with pain did they take me in. I was in the delivery suite for 26 minutes. I said I needed to push, but the midwife did not believe me,' she says. 'She broke my waters without consent. The pushing stage was done in six minutes and my child was born [with a] wound to her scalp, believed to be from the membrane hook, used when she was too far down the birth canal.' After instructing solicitors to take legal action against her NHS Trust, Keshet was inspired to study law herself, to help make a difference for others.

*

There's no doubt this kind of treatment is inexcusable, regardless of the pressures and challenges faced by midwives and other maternity staff. However, a 2020 survey by the Royal College of Midwives (RCM) does put these experiences into context, with more than 75% of midwives reporting that current levels of understaffing are 'unsafe'.

Another study, published in 2019, found that one in three doctors working in obstetrics suffers from workplace burnout – 'a condition triggered by long-term stress and overload at work, [which is] associated with emotional exhaustion, lack of empathy and connection with others, and feeling a lack of personal accomplishment'. As we've seen, this exhaustion and loss of empathy has serious safety implications for patients.

'Maternity staff are exhausted, demoralised and some of them are looking for the door. For the safety of every pregnant woman and every baby, this cannot be allowed to continue,' said Gill Walton, chief executive of the RCM. 'Midwives and maternity support workers come into the profession to provide safe, high-quality care. The legacy of underfunding and underinvestment is robbing them of that – and worse still, it's putting those women and families at risk.'

Leah Hazard is an NHS midwife and author of *Hard Pushed: A Midwife's Story*, in which she speaks candidly about the joys, pressures and challenges she faces as a midwife in a busy urban maternity hospital in Scotland. For her, the 'medical-industrial complex', where patients are seen as items on a conveyor belt rather than individual human beings, is a huge contributor to perinatal healthcare failings.

'As midwives we always hope we will provide holistic, individualised care, with the woman or birthing person at the centre of everything we do. But unfortunately, the demands of the system are such that this kind of care is very challenging to deliver,' she tells me. 'On a day-to-day basis I'm working in a unit that can often be short-staffed, with a massive caseload of women and birthing people, some of whom have incredibly complex needs, physically, emotionally and socially. You're looking at a perfect storm. As a little midwife coming into the middle of this storm, you're just one person trying to put your heart and intention into what is actually a huge machine just whirring on around you regardless.'

In a busy shift in Leah's unit, two or three midwives may see upwards of 30 women. While this isn't an excuse for poor care, she adds, it's certainly a contributing factor. 'To be absolutely clear, it's not okay ever for somebody to have something done to them without their fully informed consent. However, if you're working in a system where you feel pressurised by your superiors or colleagues, or you fear that you will face punitive measures – anything from bullying, undermining behaviour to actual disciplinary action – if your care is outside certain guidelines, I can see how that could contribute to situations where the balance of power becomes increasingly unbalanced,' Leah says. 'Unfortunately, in that kind of highly pressurised environment, the wishes of the birthing person can sometimes get lost.'

Fundamentally, she adds, it's difficult to treat people with respect and love when you are not receiving that yourself. If you as a caregiver don't feel safe and supported, it becomes much harder to make other people feel safe and supported. Clearly midwives and obstetric staff urgently need sufficient time and resources to be able to offer the high standard of patient-centred care they've been trained to give. But we also need a sea change in workplace culture to tackle the implicit biases, including racism, that Leah says are deeply embedded in some services.

*

Tinuke Awe began campaigning on Black women's maternal health after the traumatic birth of her first child. 'It was my first time, so I was quite scared anyway and didn't really know what to expect. The midwife who induced me reassured me it would take at least 24 hours,' she recalls.

'Within four or five hours I was feeling quite a lot of pain, but I was dismissed. I wasn't checked over or given any pain relief, because nobody believed I was in labour. It wasn't until hours later, when I was literally bent over double on the toilet, vomiting profusely, that my waters then broke and the midwife checked me.'

By this point, Tinuke was eight centimetres dilated – 'I will never forget the look of shock on the midwife's face,' she says – and the window of opportunity for any pain relief had been missed. Although she was finally rushed to the delivery suite, Tinuke was now too exhausted to push, her baby was back-to-back (head down, but with the baby's spine against her spine, which can make a vaginal birth more difficult) and had to be removed using forceps. Fortunately, both Tinuke and her baby were fine, but she found the experience so stressful and traumatic that she couldn't wait to get out of hospital.

Tinuke now runs a meetup group, Mums and Tea, for Black mothers and after the birth of her son heard countless stories of experiences similar to her own. When the 2018 MBRRACE report was published a year later, she was 'shocked but not surprised' to learn that Black women like her were five times more likely than white women to die in pregnancy and childbirth.

When Tinuke started digging into the data, she learned that there's been a known racial disparity in maternal mortality since at least 1991 (data on race wasn't collected prior to this), when her own mother gave birth to her. In 2020, driven by the trauma of her son's birth, and determined to ensure her newborn daughter wouldn't one day face the same risks, Tinuke teamed up with friend Clotilde Abe to launch the Five X More campaign.

Her baby girl was just four weeks old when their petition, calling on the British government to improve maternal mortality rates for Black women, took off. It gained more than 187,000 signatures, triggering a Parliamentary debate, the launch of a Race Equality Taskforce by the RCOG and a national inquiry into racial injustice in maternity care. It's an incredibly impressive legacy and an important lesson in never underestimating the power of mums.

Although the racial disparity had reduced slightly in the latest MBRRACE report, published in 2020, Black women remain four times more likely to die than their white counterparts. But, thanks to the tireless campaigning of Tinuke, Clotilde and their allies, those women's voices are now finally being heard by politicians, healthcare professionals and others with the power to effect change.

'What comes up over and over again is the feeling of not being listened to, or being dismissed by health professionals, and Black women feeling like they're being treated differently because of the colour of their skin. I've heard stories of pain relief not being given or women being sent home, because midwives didn't believe they were in labour,' Tinuke says.

Two 2022 reports – 'The Black Maternity Experiences Survey', published by Five X More, and 'Systemic racism, not broken bodies: An inquiry into racial injustice and human rights in UK maternity care', published by Birthrights – reinforce the full, shocking extent of these issues. Black, Asian and ethnic minority women describe feeling humiliated, unsafe and coerced during labour, as well as being dismissed as 'precious' or 'aggressive'. Clearly many of these experiences are not exclusive to Black and ethnic minority women, but as Tinuke says: 'The statistics speak for themselves. A lot of white women do have very traumatic birth experiences, but the fact that Black mothers only account for 4% of births in the UK yet are [four] times more likely to die is a problem.'

Of course, as consultant obstetrician and gynaecologist Dr Christine Ekechi points out, this isn't just a maternity problem: 'It's a societal problem. Maternity outcomes, and health outcomes more broadly, are just one of the ways that structural racism is manifested.' Within the maternity context, though, Christine adds, patient advocates have played a vital role in making Black women's voices and experiences heard.

As the RCOG's spokesperson on racial equality, Christine is clear that there's a lot of work to be done to tackle racial biases across all areas of women's healthcare – from improving training and education to ensuring greater diversity in senior healthcare roles. None of this can happen overnight, she says, and funding is essential to taking baby steps in the right direction. 'We are working in constrained conditions, trying to deliver excellent care with reducing resources,' she explains. 'NHS Trusts need more people and more resources – especially if we're asking them to be ever more cognisant of racial inequalities, and to put measures in place to try and address them.'

Christine is hopeful that a focus on maternal mortality can help to break the cycle of racial disparity, but she also believes it's just the tip of the iceberg. 'If a baby is born into a cycle of inequality and we don't address the disparities, those disparities continue,' she says. 'Maternal mortality in the UK is low, but everybody should be able to benefit from that equally. Maternal morbidity – where people are very sick or injured in a way that impairs their life – is equally important and we see the same racial disparity there. It's vital we acknowledge that, too, and that we tackle health inequalities throughout Black people's lives.'

*

Regardless of their pregnancy and birth experience, the postnatal period is rife with challenges for all new parents. As Hysterical Women contributor Steph Cullen says, 'Everyone wants to hold the baby, but who holds the mum?' In the midst of juggling the demands of a newborn, too many women and birthing people again find their own health overlooked and dismissed – or, as I'll explore in the next chapter, find concerns about their baby's health dismissed as the irrational panic of an overly anxious new mum.

Of first-time mothers who give birth vaginally, 90% experience some kind of perineal tear, graze or cut (episiotomy). Most of these are minor and heal quickly after birth, but 3.5% are classed as third and fourth-degree tears, or obstetric anal sphincter injuries (OASI).

A shockingly high number of mums suffer with postnatal incontinence, with at least one in three affected by urinary incontinence and one in 10 affected by some form of anal incontinence at six weeks postpartum. As their child is nearing the end of primary school 10 years later, one in five are still experiencing urinary incontinence and 3% faecal incontinence.

Similarly, at 12 and 20 years postnatally, almost a third will have symptoms of pelvic organ prolapse – where one or more of the bowel, bladder or uterus slip down and bulge into the vagina – even after just one vaginal birth. This, according to the British Society of Urogynaecology, is rarely seen in women who have not been pregnant. If men were leaking piss and poo at such a staggering rate, it would (rightly) be viewed as a health crisis, but, when it comes to mothers, incontinence and prolapse are too often treated as inevitable.

One particularly horrifying story, shared on Hysterical Women by Chantelle, describes waiting three years and eight months for surgery to fix an obstetric anal sphincter injury, after her 'beautiful wrecking ball' of a third baby 'popped out of my arse'. 'This exact operation would have been done on the day of birth if they'd given me a rectal examination and realised the extent of the injury there and then,' she tells me. Instead, she was left with full bowel incontinence for the best part of four years, which took a devastating toll on Chantelle's relationship, family life and career. Meanwhile, doctors offered her the futile reassurance that, 'sometimes these things happen'.

Luce Brett, author of *PMSL: Or How I Literally Pissed Myself Laughing and Survived the Last Taboo to Tell the Tale,* writes movingly and candidly about her experiences with postnatal urinary incontinence. 'Lots of people perpetuated the lie – women themselves and doctors – that incontinence is a normal thing post-childbirth,' Luce says. 'I felt drenched in these lies.'

Research suggests new mothers suffering from incontinence are almost twice as likely to develop postnatal depression, and Luce describes feeling almost suicidally depressed at times. Yet she also tells me about being dismissed as 'just another stressed mum', as if the misery of regularly wetting yourself is part and parcel of the sacrifice all mothers should make, selflessly and unflinchingly, for their offspring. For this reason, *PMSL* is more than just a deeply personal memoir to Luce; it's also a feminist manifesto for change. It's one mother's campaign for healthcare professionals to rethink postnatal care, incontinence and pelvic health for all birthing people.

One healthcare professional fighting for exactly that is pelvic physiotherapist Elaine Miller, co-founder of campaign group Pelvic Roar, whose comedy show *Gusset Grippers* uses humour to tackle incontinence taboos. 'The problem with birth is it's really not a good bit of evolutionary design. You have to get a very large object through a very small channel and leave both unscathed,' she explains.

In that sense, Elaine adds, it's inevitable that pregnancy puts your pelvic floor at risk – even if you have a C-section. But, she says, 'Although it's common, it's not normal to have injuries that interfere with what you do with the rest of your life; you don't need to put up with it.'

Except for the most severe birth injuries, virtually all postnatal pelvic floor issues can be solved or even prevented by pelvic physiotherapy and regular pelvic floor exercises. According to Elaine, around a third of the women she sees in clinic only ever come to her once. All most postnatal parents need, she explains, is a bit of basic pelvic floor education and reassurance, and then the vast majority can manage their symptoms by themselves.

It should be this easy, but torn perineums and weakened pelvic floors get forgotten. 'Often women themselves don't have a good handle on what the problem actually is. They're so overwhelmed and exhausted that it's really challenging to engage with their own healthcare when they've got young children,' Elaine says.

A more proactive approach from GPs, midwives and health visitors would be the ideal, Elaine says, to probe and check in on any potential issues that frazzled new parents might forget or feel too ashamed to mention. One significant step towards addressing this came in 2021, with the announcement of 14 NHS pelvic health clinics opening across England, bringing together doctors, midwives and physiotherapists to support those struggling with pelvic floor issues.

A survey published by MUTU System, an app-based pre-and post-natal exercise and support programme, confirms how urgently needed this service is, with 91% of respondents saying they weren't given enough advice during pregnancy about postnatal recovery. Eighty-four per cent went on to experience some kind of postnatal health issue, but 89% felt unprepared with techniques to aid their recovery.

As a champion of post-birth vaginas, Luce also hears plenty of stories about health professionals dismissing incontinence, prolapse and postnatal sexual dysfunction as a natural part of being a mother. 'It's as if being broken is a price we should all happily pay for having had children; as if it is 'enough' to have had a child,' she says. 'You can see the difference when you compare it to the discourse about Viagra and problems with penises. With childbirth we have such levels of ignorance and shame, so those stories have been lost to silence.' It is precisely this silence that allows poor practice to continue unchecked and unscrutinised, keeping neglected patient groups conveniently out of sight and out of mind.

*

Self-advocacy can be even more fraught for trans, queer and non-binary birthing parents, who face their own unique set of challenges in perinatal healthcare. Not being a woman, in a system that's so overwhelmingly set up for women, would be a challenge anyway, but it is particularly difficult against the backdrop of the virulent transphobia we've already observed.

Jacob Stokoe is a trans masculine 'papa' who, at the time of writing, has a three-year-old daughter and is six months pregnant with his second baby. Jacob has been supporting birthing people for years and is due to begin training as a postnatal doula shortly after the birth of his second child. For him, many aspects of perinatal healthcare have triggered a lot of gender dysphoria. Much of this came in the form of what Jacob calls 'indirect misgendering' – the 'relentless' language of 'women' and 'mothers' that consistently appears on posters, in letters, emails and online resources about pregnancy and birth. Invariably, he points out, this is unnecessary. 'A poster saying, "If you're here for a scan, make sure you've got a full bladder" feels much warmer and more inviting than, "All pregnant women must have a full bladder," as well as being accidentally inclusive,' he says.

'Transphobia in the UK is rife and it's spreading. As a community we're fearful and exhausted, so these are unnecessary stressors for those of us growing our families in the middle of it. I don't think cis people realise how physically painful misgendering is, in a way that's really difficult to explain unless you've experienced it,' Jacob says. 'There were years of my life when my deadname [birth name] and my previous pronouns were weaponised against me, deliberately and repeatedly.'

In the postnatal period too, he recalls grappling with his identity as a birthing parent. 'I felt like I was everything a mother was, but not female, and the word 'mother' felt very triggering to me. My daughter had been part of my body and I'd been through this life-changing event of growing and birthing her, but my role was completely invisible,' he says. In the end the family settled on 'Papa', as a way of differentiating Jacob from his husband ('Daddy'), but he describes the experience as one of what he calls 'postnatal dysphoria'. This also manifested in difficult and complex emotions around chest-feeding. While not exclusive to trans parents – breast-feeding aversion is well documented among cis mothers – this did come with the added baggage of gender dysphoria, on top of the hormonal changes and postnatal depression he also experienced.

Jacob feels he's been lucky, for the most part, in his interactions with healthcare professionals, but he's all too aware of the issues many trans parents face. 'It's really obvious when someone hasn't worked with a trans person before or had any training, and that makes a big difference,' he says. His first community midwife fell into this camp – uninformed and clumsily misgendering, in a 'well-meaning but rubbish' rather than 'actively transphobic' way. The biggest issue, though, was her attempt at gatekeeping his birth choices when he expressed a desire for a home birth.

Fortunately, Jacob was able to get a referral via his GP and spent the rest of his pregnancy and birth under the care of two midwives from the home birth team. 'They were fantastic,' he says. 'It was a learning curve for them, but they listened and worked hard to make sure I felt safe and comfortable. I've been really lucky.' This, he says, is largely down to a combination of privileges – being able to self-advocate articulately, having a good support network, being white, masculine-passing and having a middle-class husband.

The privilege of being perceived as male is a particularly interesting double-edged sword. 'I've witnessed the kind of talking down to and infantilising that happens to women and femme-presenting people in healthcare. You see that even more so when people are pregnant. There's this sense that you're on these river rapids and you don't get a say in which direction you're going; you've just got to get down them, be a "good girl" and get this baby out, regardless of what it does to you,' he says. 'As a masculine person, when I go to a doctor's appointment they see a man, so I'm not infantilised in the same way that I've witnessed and experienced myself before my transition.'

Jacob is passionate about continuing to advocate on behalf of other trans birthing parents who aren't so lucky. Besides formally training as a doula, Jacob plans to continue this work as one quarter of the Queer Parenting Partnership – alongside midwives Kay and Maeve, and doula Kim. Within this team, co-founders Kim and Kay focus on providing support for queer people making families, while Maeve and Jacob provide training to birth professionals.

'Continuity of carer is particularly key for trans and non-binary birthing parents. It's really scary meeting someone you don't know as a trans person, especially when you're in the vulnerable position of giving birth. You never know how a new person is going to be with you and whether you'll have to spend a significant amount of your limited appointment time explaining who you are, what your pronouns are, or being on edge waiting for the slip up,' he says.

The broader context of transphobia again adds to this needless anxiety. In 2021 Brighton and Sussex Hospitals Trust was at the receiving end of a backlash against their decision to incorporate gender-neutral language – such as 'birthing parent' and 'chest-feeding' – into their perinatal healthcare services. The Trust was accused of 'erasing' women and mothers from their services, despite making it perfectly clear they were doing no such thing. 'We are taking a gender-additive approach to the language used to describe our services, [which] means using gender-neutral language alongside the language of womanhood, in order to ensure that everyone is represented and included,' the Trust's policy document stated.

'Every step we take forward stirs up new waves of transphobia,' Jacob says. 'Thankfully, many individuals in birth work are fully supportive of trans and non-binary birthing people – or they want to be, which is where our training comes in – but we need to find a way to utilise these positive voices to drown out the negative.'

This is particularly true as the number of trans parents giving birth continues to rise. Data on non-female birthing parents is not centrally collected in the UK but, according to research from the Improving Trans Experiences of Maternity

Services (ITEMS) project, 54 trans people gave birth in England between 2016 and 2020, compared to just two between 1996 and 2000.

Jacob believes increasing visibility of parents like him and journalist Freddy McConnell – whose pregnancy is documented in 2019 film *Seahorse* – will empower more trans and gender-nonconforming individuals to pursue pregnancy for themselves. 'Many trans people of my generation were told testosterone would make us infertile and we should have a hysterectomy. It took a long time for me to learn that I could come off testosterone and get pregnant. Younger generations have much more knowledge and information about their choices,' he says.

'I've seen much more interest in the three years since I had my daughter and that makes advocating for inclusive birthing spaces so much more necessary. I'm not going to use that waiting room again after this baby's born, but I know other people like me will use it.' We also know that the current way of doing things isn't working for women either. Vast swathes of birthing people are already being let down, dismissed and forgotten during pregnancy, birth and the postnatal period. Transforming services to be safe and inclusive for everyone who brings new life into the world is surely a positive and vital goal.

Indeed, as Jacob adds, most of the things that are good for trans people are good for everybody – particularly birthing people who have experienced previous traumas. 'It's all about recognising the autonomy of an individual and the language that individual uses for themselves,' he says. Regardless of your gender, it's clear that choice and autonomy throughout pregnancy and birth reduce the risk of trauma – something Jacob's particularly passionate about because of the number of cis women he knows who have been left traumatised by their experiences. By making birth services inclusive and tailored to individuals, he says, the 'river rapids' of childbirth can be shaped to the path that each birthing person wants to take.

★

Perinatal mental health is, of course, intimately wrapped up in all these other experiences – from the emotional impact of Charlotte's hyperemesis and Luce's incontinence, to Tinuke and Keshet's traumatic births, and Jacob's postnatal dysphoria. But if the physical health of birthing people is seen as secondary to that of their foetus, their mental health invariably finds itself shoved even further to the bottom of the pile.

'Pregnancy and birth are a uniquely vulnerable time. When things go well, people feel heard, respected, validated and supported. When they don't go well, they can feel alone, very frightened and very out of control,' says Dr Rebecca Moore, a perinatal psychiatrist and co-founder of Make Birth Better, which campaigns on reducing birth trauma and helps both parents and professionals find support.

'Stigma around perinatal mental healthcare is huge still, particularly in some communities, because women understandably feel worried about being judged or shamed, or that their child might be taken away from them,' Rebecca says. 'It may be difficult for some women to navigate services, because of complex needs, if English is not their first language, or because of a fear and lack of trust in the health service. It can also sometimes be really frustrating as a patient – and I've been there myself – to have to chase and lead your own care. That's hard anyway, but it's really, really difficult if you've got a two-week-old baby and you feel knackered,' she adds.

During pregnancy too, many expectant parents feel ashamed about struggling with anxiety or depression at a time when they're expected to feel happy and excited about their impending arrival. For Lauren, who suffered from antenatal depression, that shame was compounded by the unhelpful attitudes she encountered from her GP and midwife. 'It was all very much, "Don't worry, you'll get over it. As soon as you hold the baby, you'll be fine,"' she recalls.

Laura Cooke suffered from tokophobia – an intense fear of childbirth – and self-referred to an NHS mental health support service while pregnant with her first child. By the time she'd been through two telephone assessments, Laura was told – just into her third trimester – that she was, in her words, 'too pregnant' for mental health support.

For Black mums, these barriers to maternal mental health support are aggravated even further by cultural stigmas and racist stereotyping. Sandra Igwe, founder of the Motherhood Group, which focuses on sharing and supporting the Black maternal experience, and co-chair of the national inquiry into racial injustice in maternity care, says, 'Mental health in the Black community is still only just being spoken about. Our parents don't necessarily believe it's something Black people go through.' In fact, she points out, Black mothers are more likely than white mothers to experience postnatal depression or anxiety, but much less likely to receive treatment.

She believes the racist myth of the 'strong, independent Black woman' contributes to Black mothers not getting the support they need. 'When we do speak out, our views and our words are dismissed. To get support, a lot of the time it feels like you have to be on the upper end of the spectrum, suffering from psychosis or in danger of physically harming your baby,' Sandra says.

NHS England has, Rebecca points out, invested significantly in improving perinatal mental healthcare over the last decade, and services are much better than they once were. But there remains a broader issue around NHS mental health services being dangerously overstretched and under-resourced. 'It's frustrating at times because we, as mental healthcare professionals, can't offer care to all and there are often long waiting lists for therapy,' she says. 'The pressure on services is such that it is so often only the women with very severe illness who get rapid, bespoke care. It feels like you're almost waiting for people to get more and more unwell before the care actually kicks in, which seems completely the wrong way round.'

Perhaps unsurprisingly given this struggle to access support during pregnancy, many women find their symptoms continue into the postnatal period. Research by the National Childbirth Trust (NCT) shows that half of new mums experience mental health difficulties during pregnancy or within the first year after birth. Despite this, one in four new mothers are not asked about their mental health at their six-week check, with 85% saying the appointment focused mainly or equally on the baby's health at the expense of their own. For Lauren, postnatal depression culminated in a suicide attempt when her baby was three months old – at which point she was finally referred for therapy. But how much harm could have been prevented if only Lauren had been properly supported sooner?

YOUR PERINATAL TOOLKIT

Clearly the onus shouldn't be on vulnerable people to fight for the care they need at any stage of their perinatal journey, but speaking out can be useful if you feel able to. 'Remember that you have the right to be given evidence-based information and to have a two-way discussion about all reasonable options,' say Maria Booker and Jo Rhys-Davies, respectively programmes director and advice officer at Birthrights. When it comes to birth choices, they add, don't feel pressured to make decisions immediately – you can often say: 'Thank you for that information, I will let you know my decision at our next appointment.'

If you feel you're not being listened to during birth, Maria and Jo recommend saying something immediately, using clear language like, 'Stop,' 'I don't consent,' 'I don't feel listened to' or 'You're hurting me.' You're also entitled to ask for a few minutes alone with your partner or supporters to gather your thoughts, or to speak to the senior manager on call. Equally, if you don't feel able to advocate for yourself, ask your birth partner to step in or contact the hospital's PALS. Of course, all of these can be difficult to think of in the moment, so it's a good idea to have this discussion with your birth partner beforehand, as part of your preparations for labour.

Most importantly, remember that any bad care you receive is never your fault – even if you don't feel able to speak out at the time. You can always make a complaint after the fact, so your experience goes on record and can help to inform Trust policy going forwards. Googling your local Maternity Voices Partnership (MVP) in England or Maternity Services Liaison Committee (MSLC) in the rest of the UK is a great place to start.

During pregnancy and the postnatal period, you can also ask a trusted GP or midwife to signpost or refer you to any relevant local support services, whether that's perinatal mental healthcare, pelvic physiotherapy, breast- or chest-feeding support, or local parent and baby groups. Make the most of the wealth of supportive online peer support communities, too, and remember that you're not alone with whatever you're going through.

Resources
- AIMS (Association for Improving Maternity Services) – aims.org.uk
- Birthrights – birthrights.org.uk
- Birth Trauma Association – birthtraumaassociation. org.uk
- Breastfeeding Aversion – breastfeedingaversion.com
- Five X More – fivexmore.com
- La Leche League (breast-feeding support) – laleche.org.uk
- Make Birth Better – makebirthbetter.org
- Maternal Mental Health Alliance – maternalmentalh ealthalliance.org
- MASIC Foundation (support after birth injuries) – masic.org.uk
- Miscarriage Association – miscarriageassociation.org.uk
- Mums and Tea (for Black mothers) – mumsandtea.com
- National Childbirth Trust – nct.org.uk
- Not Morning Sickness campaign – notmorningsickness .com

- PANDAS Foundation (perinatal mental health support) – pandasfoundation.org.uk
- Pelvic Roar – pelvicroar.org
- Positive Birth Movement – positivebirthmovement.org
- Pregnancy Sickness Support – pregnancysicknesssupport.org.uk
- Prosperitys (for Black and south Asian mothers) – instagram.com/_prosperitys
- Queer Birth Club – queerbirthclub.co.uk
- Sands (stillbirth and neonatal death) – sands.org.uk
- Squeezy App (pelvic floor support) – squeezyapp.com
- The Motherhood Group (for Black mothers) – themotherhoodgroup.com
- The Queer Parenting Partnership – parentingqueer.co.uk
- Tommy's Midwives – tommys.org

9

'Death means we believe you now': Neurotic mothers in healthcare

Sadly, the mistreatment of mothers is not exclusive to perinatal care. It persists in the doctor's office long after teenage acne and period pains have taken the place of neonatal jaundice and croup. Yet from the moment of conception – at least in the eyes of certain healthcare professionals – women who give birth take on the mantle of 'neurotic mother', with all capacity for rational thought wiped out by their all-consuming love and concern for their precious offspring.

'We live with this narrative whereby maternal self-sacrifice is expected of women,' Clare Murphy says. But when the shit hits the fan, no matter how much they've given up of their own lives, bodies and health, mothers' knowledge, experience and expertise are still so easily dismissed as not to be trusted.

In the previous chapter I mentioned Clare Norton, who lost her daughter Lara after she was born breech and not breathing in 1995. The following year, her third daughter Merryn was born, and at six months old Clare took her to hospital, concerned about how poorly her baby was. Staff assured her there was nothing to worry about, but Clare refused to be fobbed off and sent home. When Merryn was eventually transferred to a children's hospital, she was diagnosed with a very bad case of bronchiolitis and kept in for a week. A nurse in the first hospital had written 'over-anxious mother' in Merryn's notes, but – for neither the first nor the last time – Clare's maternal instincts had been spot-on.

As a health journalist I hear dozens of women's stories, but few have ever haunted me quite like the harrowing tale of what came next for Clare and Merryn. Two decades later, in 2017, 21-year-old Merryn Crofts became the second person in the UK to have her death officially attributed to severe ME, the complex chronic illness that primarily affects women, but which, as I mention in chapter 4, some doctors don't even believe exists.

For years before that, both Merryn and Clare had fought against doctors insisting her illness was all in her head – that it was anxiety, or an eating disorder, and that her physical symptoms could be cured by psychological therapies. This culminated in an accusation of fabricated and induced illness (FII), previously known as Munchausen by proxy, when medical staff claimed Clare had actually caused her daughter's illness.

Clare contributed a post for Hysterical Women in March 2019, almost two years after Merryn's death. I have thought about her final words on a regular basis ever since: 'For me, it's reminiscent of the witch trials, where drowning meant you were innocent,' she wrote. 'Death means we believe you now.'

Those five words have stuck with me and become a kind of driving force for Hysterical Women. Merryn's story is rare, of course, and the very worst-case scenario for ME patients. But how many more women have to die before doctors will believe their accounts of what's going on in their own bodies?

While Merryn's story is devastating and tragic in and of itself, I was also struck by doctors' treatment of Clare and how much it chimed with other stories I'd heard. Another guest writer, Emily Ryalls, described how she and her mother, in their quest for a diagnosis, had been 'reduced [by doctors] to "over-anxious mother and hypochondriac teenage daughter."'

Clare seemed to fit that same hysterical mythology of the over-anxious, over-protective, neurotic mother figure. It's a stereotype we're all familiar with: the perpetually worried and indulgent mum, jumping to their little darling's every whim, rushing them to the doctor at the slightest sniffle and constantly looking for signs that something's wrong.

More recently, it was exactly this stereotype that Lui Sit applied to her own behaviour when, at just a few months old, her daughter Molly developed a persistent cough. After repeated trips to her unconcerned family GP, Lui, like so many women, began to question whether her own judgement was at fault. Was she just a hysterical first-time mum, unable to cope and wasting the GP's time too often?

'As we leave the building, I wonder if it is lack of sleep and parenting experience that is turning me into a zealous mother, oversensitive to every sniffle that Molly emits,' she writes. 'I lecture myself to adopt the stance of the GP and ignore the niggling feeling inside. After all, I am a brand-new mother, what do I know?'

Unable to ignore the niggle for long, however, Lui persisted. After a year and countless GP visits, she and Molly were finally referred to a specialist. 'He speaks to me as an equal and actively listens. His comments are insightful and concise, and he answers my many questions with patience and no condescension,' Lui recalls with gratitude. More importantly, he provided the vindication she had been searching for, diagnosing Molly with breathing issues caused by mild bulbar palsy, a neurological condition. 'Something *was* wrong – despite many medical professionals insisting otherwise,' Lui writes.

*

From her earliest years, Clare recalls Merryn as a bundle of energy who would dance rather than walk into a room. But when Merryn was 15, she developed debilitating fatigue, along with a host of other symptoms, including swelling in her face, hands and feet, difficulty breathing and nausea. Clare knew something wasn't right. Within months, Merryn had deteriorated drastically – from a vibrant, sociable teenager to a seriously ill young woman who was reliant on a wheelchair.

'We had to move her bedroom downstairs and get her a commode. As a mother, it was terrifying to see her change so quickly like that,' Clare says. 'I felt helpless. You'd do anything to protect your children or take away any pain they're going through. I felt like I should be fixing this, but I couldn't.'

When the family GP insisted on Merryn being referred to Child and Adolescent Mental Health Services (CAMHS) for mental health treatment, she willingly went along – with the intention of proving him wrong. 'She'd been to CAMHS for mental health problems before, when she was younger, so we didn't have anything against talking about mental health. But we knew that wasn't the issue in this case. When she saw CAMHS they confirmed that it was absolutely a physical issue,' Clare says.

Despite this, during the numerous hospital admissions and doctors' visits that followed, healthcare professionals continued to suggest it was a mental health problem. It took a year, and the family paying for a private consultation, to get Merryn diagnosed with ME and referred to see a specialist ME consultant on the NHS, albeit one outside their local area. Meanwhile, Clare had given up work and was caring for her daughter full-time.

As Merryn's condition worsened it began to affect her stomach and swallowing, and she lost weight rapidly. Despite her ME diagnosis and Merryn's own desire to have a feeding tube fitted, gastroenterology specialists suggested she was suffering from anorexia. 'We had meeting after meeting and eventually they agreed to fit a feeding tube, but it was yet another fight,' Clare says.

By this time, Merryn had severe photosensitivity and noise sensitivity. She had to wear sunglasses and noise-cancelling headphones a lot of the time, even indoors, and speaking had become difficult. But doctors weren't happy when Clare insisted on staying during Merryn's procedure. 'I think they thought I was just an over-protective mother, but I wasn't leaving. I always had to stay with her now when she went into hospital, because she just couldn't communicate herself and I knew what she needed,' she explains.

Merryn's surgery was to fit a percutaneous endoscopic gastrostomy (known as a PEG) – a feeding tube inserted directly into the stomach. It's a traumatic operation, which Clare later learned is usually done under general anaesthetic in under 18s, but 17-year-old Merryn was simply sedated. 'One of the side-effects of ME for Merryn was that medication just didn't touch her. She'd had the sedation and she was saying, "I can still feel everything,"' Clare says, her voice trembling at the memory. Throughout the procedure, Clare recalls watching in horror, begging healthcare staff to stop, as her teenage daughter screamed in agony. Apparently unmoved by Clare and Merryn's protestations, they continued. After surgery, when Clare rushed to have words with the doctor, his response was: 'Get out of my way, you stupid woman, I've got to go and save somebody's life.'

I find it unspeakably horrifying to think of any healthcare professional continuing to work through the screams of their teenage patient. But how does it come to this? The God complex apparent in this doctor's words perhaps goes some way towards explaining it. I don't believe doctors go into the profession actively intending to do harm, but I can see how the power and status that comes with saving lives could lead to the kind of egos the profession is still known for.

Equally, I can see how the horrors that doctors deal with every day could leave them desensitised to a certain amount of pain and suffering. But could a doctor really be cocksure enough to believe, in the face of such visceral evidence, that the girl in front of him can't feel a thing? Maybe, if the alternative is accepting that what's worked for previous patients might not work for them all. That medicine, in other words, might not be as infallible as he's been taught to believe.

On the Sunday, after two days recovering in hospital, Clare was expecting to take Merryn home. That's when a nurse dropped the bombshell: a safeguarding referral had been made to social services. Clare had been accused of causing Merryn's illness, lying about her symptoms and answering for Merryn instead of letting her daughter speak. 'Thankfully, when the social worker came out to see us she was brilliant and said the referral was absolute rubbish. But we could so easily have had a social worker who believed all of that,' she says.

After her death in 2017, Merryn's inquest concluded that ME was the cause. Clare says, 'Merryn would love that vindication because it was like them saying, "We believe you," after all those times when she wasn't believed, when she even questioned herself. She used to say to me, "Do you think it's all in my head?" and I said, "Never. Never ever, because I know you." It's vindication for that.'

It's a bittersweet vindication, one that doesn't bring Merryn back, or answer Clare's many unanswerable questions about if or how things could have been different. I finish our call fighting back tears of my own and in absolute awe of the way Clare has continued to fight for Merryn's legacy under the weight of a grief I can't even begin to imagine. She keeps telling me how strong, brave and determined Merryn was and – although Clare doesn't seem to recognise it herself – it's clear that's a trait she inherited from her mother.

*

Mothers exist in a weird cultural limbo: at times revered and held up as paragons of selfless, self-sacrificing unconditional love and care; in the next breath reviled as the source of so many of society's ills. Every choice a mother makes is scrutinised in minute detail, whether she's a single mum (feckless), a working mum (negligent) or a stay-at-home mum (dependent). I've even caught myself doing it – wondering how the mothers of so many adult men still allow their sons to leave home without basic life skills like cooking and cleaning. What about the examples set by their fathers, who in the vast majority of cases get off scot-free for their contributions to parenting? Even the phrase 'daddy issues' is used to shame women, not the fathers who failed them.

When it comes to women's everyday lives, parenting remains one of the most obvious bastions of gender inequality. This isn't exclusive to health, but seeps into virtually every aspect of professional, personal and domestic life. Mothers are expected to do everything, know everything and be everything to everyone. But they're also belittled, as in Clare's case, as 'stupid women'. When it really counts, they are seen as 'just a mum'; neurotic, overprotective, making a fuss. Their maternal instinct, intuition and intimate knowledge of their own children become meaningless in the face of those who see themselves as the real experts.

In most nuclear, heterosexual families, the mother is almost invariably the parent who takes time off work when their child is sick, who accompanies them to appointments, collects their prescriptions, warms their soup and mops their brow. Yet countless girls and young women tell me doctors only took them seriously once their dad got involved – or that doctors consistently dismissed their mum's opinion as much as their own.

Like many teenagers, 13-year-old Robyn Atcheson was accompanied to the local surgery by her mum when her periods caused debilitating pain, heavy bleeding and fainting during school. 'For years both my mum and I were dismissed as hysterical women. Doctors kept trying to palm me off, believing I didn't understand what periods were meant to be like. I knew from talking to other girls my age that not everyone suffered like this, but I was met with complete dismissal and disbelief,' Robyn says.

By the time she eventually got a diagnosis, 10 years later, endometriosis had caused permanent damage to her bladder and bowel, for which she still requires treatment. 'There was so much sexism in doctors' responses,' she adds. 'My mum had experienced endometriosis herself – we both knew the symptoms – but doctors said she was projecting onto me; that she'd put the idea in my head and I was trying to copy her; I was overdramatic and attention-seeking; it was all in our heads.'

The invasive nature of the laparoscopic surgery currently required to formally diagnose endometriosis does, of course, present ethical issues when the patient is in her teens. As consultant paediatrician Dr Keir Shiels says, 'Any doctor would be struck off if they recommended opening up every teenage girl who presented with painful periods' – highlighting Endometriosis UK's point about the urgent need for a more straightforward diagnostic test.

However, Keir adds, 'There is a huge difficulty, which we don't talk enough about in medicine. How much empathy and understanding do most male doctors – and even female doctors who haven't experienced it themselves – have about problems relating to periods?' In Robyn's case, there was no attempt to manage her symptoms in the meantime, or to rule out other causes; just a flat-out denial of her pain.

Robyn is now in her early 30s, but her mother Jacqui Lowry still accompanies her to every appointment. Looking back on her daughter's teenage periods, Jacqui says she knew Robyn's symptoms weren't normal, but doctors refused to acknowledge her experience and expertise. 'It was like hitting my head against a brick wall, saying, "Listen to me, this is what she has – I've been through it,"' she recalls.

Nearly a decade on from her diagnosis, Robyn still lives with the chronic pain of endometriosis, and the added bladder and bowel complications that might have been avoided if she had been diagnosed and treated earlier. 'There's nothing I can do apart from sit and hold her while she's crying, and plug her heated pad in for her,' Jacqui says. 'I would do anything in the world to take the pain away from her.'

*

Besides Clare, Lui and Jacqui, the other 'neurotic mother' I've been most struck by is Caron Ryalls, whose daughter Emily I mentioned earlier. A no-nonsense, straight-talking Yorkshire woman, Caron describes herself as 'battling healthcare politics, the patriarchy and the ironing pile in my front room.' There are many parallels between Emily's story and Merryn's, except that Emily is still here to tell it herself, alongside Caron.

Looking back now, Caron says, her maternal instincts were first dismissed very early on when, like Merryn, Emily became seriously ill as a baby. After two weeks of being repeatedly brushed off by the family GP, Caron recalls bursting into tears on the phone to her own mother. 'My mum said, "If you think there's something wrong, take her to A&E and refuse to leave until it's sorted. You're the only one who will fight for her." So that's what I did,' she explains.

Emily was admitted to hospital for several days and bounced back after being given fluids and anti-viral medication, but doctors continued to insist it had just been a virus. It wasn't until Emily became ill as a teenager and Caron applied for her medical notes that she discovered Emily had actually been suffering from pneumonia.

Looking back on her childhood, Emily says her whole life centred around sport and competitive dancing. She was athletic, active, full of life, as well as being very academic. When she became ill, suddenly developing extreme fatigue and dizziness during her second year of secondary school, it was a huge change – but doctors insisted this was 'just how teenage girls are.' She says, 'It was very frustrating because I knew myself and my mum knew me. I wasn't just a lethargic teenager who couldn't be bothered to get out of bed. That's not who I am.'

On one occasion, Caron describes seeing a male GP with Emily, who was suffering from such joint pain in her knees that she could hardly walk. 'The GP's manner was nice and I really felt like he was trying to help, but what he actually said was just awful. He kept saying over and over that the mind is a very powerful part of your body and can create physical symptoms that feel very real, but there's nothing actually wrong with her. It was classic gaslighting,' she says. 'It just felt like, for so many years, everyone was talking at me and telling me what they thought was wrong,' Emily adds. 'But no one, in all those years, had actually done the tests and really listened to what I was saying. It just felt like a waste of time.'

In the meantime, Caron had sacrificed her own business and taken on the new full-time job of caring for Emily and intently researching her symptoms, while her husband worked three different jobs to make up for the loss of her wage. Eventually, she landed on PoTS – postural orthostatic tachycardia syndrome – an abnormal increase in heart rate that occurs after standing up or sitting down, which seemed to fit. But Emily's paediatrician was particularly resistant to what he saw as the mother's interference, laughing when presented with her hefty folder of research.

Emily describes the atmosphere in those appointments as 'toxic', with Caron banished to the back of the room, facing the back of the paediatrician's head and forbidden from speaking. 'I wanted Mum to be able to advocate for me when I wasn't well enough to say what I wanted to say, but she wasn't allowed,' Emily recalls. Instead, she describes holding 'strategic meetings' with her mother before each appointment, planning in meticulous detail how to get their point across in a way that couldn't be twisted or used against them. 'We really had to pander to his ego and overanalyse everything I was going to say,' she says.

I'm particularly struck by Emily's final comment as something I recognise from my own experience. As women, pandering to male egos is something we learn to do habitually from a young age. If it's not your doctor, it's your arrogant male colleague or your cocky classmate who has to be right at any cost. We're socialised not to challenge, to put our own ideas across in a way that allows him to believe he thought of them first and to laugh at his terrible jokes. If we dare to step out of line and assert ourselves, we're 'punished' like Caron and Clare – labelled as 'bossy', 'difficult' or 'interfering', or worse, silenced and reported to social services.

In the patient-doctor power dynamic, there's a particular conflict between two very different, but very valid, forms of knowledge: years of lived experience vs years of medical training and textbook knowledge. But, while patients are expected to submit to their doctor's medical expertise, there's very little recognition that patients are the experts on their own, and their children's, bodies. Instead, there seems to be a real reluctance among some doctors to admit that they don't have all the answers. To Caron, her thick file of research was a labour of love – a proactive attempt to collaborate with doctors in their common purpose of making Emily better. To Emily's paediatrician, it was easier to dismiss her as an 'interfering mother' than swallow his pride and accept that her expertise might actually complement his own.

Fortunately, through further research, Caron located a PoTS specialist an hour's drive away, and one of their more supportive GPs arranged an urgent referral. Sure enough, two and a half years after her symptoms began, Emily was diagnosed with PoTS. Another mother vindicated, but should it really have been such a battle?

*

Although Emily and Caron were always 'strategic' about toeing the line, they do tell me the threat of being reported to social services hung over them continually – particularly as they were aware of other families in similar positions who had been. It's clearly a hugely delicate issue for healthcare professionals too. How do you fulfil your duty of care and identify any genuine risks of harm, while also challenging your own biases and trusting the women in front of you?

Dr Emma Reinhold is a former GP, a researcher and a clinical advisor on complex, multi-system chronic conditions, including PoTS, EDS (Ehlers-Danlos Syndrome, which she suffers from herself), MCAS (mast cell activation syndrome) and the wastebasket diagnosis of 'medically unexplained symptoms' (MUS). She also has an interest in considering where there may be false accusations of FII against mothers of children with these difficult-to-diagnose conditions.

There are, of course, challenges for any doctors dealing with young patients and their parents, but, Emma says, GPs and paediatricians are well trained to deal with these different dynamics. 'You'll always try to start off by engaging the child and asking them what's been happening. With older children and teenagers, you should also offer them the opportunity to kick their parent out of the consultation, because they have every right to see you without their parent present,' she explains.

On some occasions the child will take the lead, she adds, while in other situations they might not want to speak to you because they're too shy or – like Merryn and Emily – don't feel able to advocate for themselves. In those instances, Emma says, GPs will default to the parent. It's a challenging dynamic, she acknowledges, but one that's bread and butter for any family doctor.

So why do these accusations seem to happen so frequently in chronic illness circles? Emma believes much of the problem begins with doctors' ignorance about the conditions, as we explored in chapter 4, and their failure to make a correct diagnosis. 'If you haven't got a diagnosis, children with fluctuating, multisystem symptoms are likely to be labelled with "perplexing presentations", which is the paediatric equivalent of MUS. Current child protection training is that any "perplexing presentation" should be considered a safeguarding concern,' she explains. Just as medically unexplained symptoms in adults are too often dismissed as 'psychosomatic', she believes there's a tendency in paediatrics to view 'perplexing presentations' in children as fabricated, exaggerated or induced by the parent, rather than simply 'not yet diagnosed.'

This, she says, is made worse by a paranoia resulting from cases like the death of Baby P. 'Every single time there's a case where a child dies at the hands of their parent, the blame game happens and healthcare professionals get more and more anxious. For us as professionals, the safest option for our reputation is to default to the highest level of safeguarding investigation, refer everything, and to disregard the impact and the harm of that investigation to families,' Emma says.

'We're also told in safeguarding training not to trust parents; that malicious parents will lie and other parents are well-meaning but overly anxious, and exaggerate their children's symptoms. These two ends of the spectrum have really been conflated, so all of these families are taken down the same safeguarding pathway,' she adds. 'Obviously there are genuinely people who harm their children. It's pretty rare, but it absolutely does happen and we have to accept that, believe it and keep it in the back of our minds. But then you also have parents who maybe make a little bit more of something than you might think is objective and parents who are really, genuinely concerned because their child has got unexplained symptoms and they can't help.'

From Emma's perspective, though, as a woman with EDS and a mother of two children, many of the criteria for accusing a parent of FII are exactly the type of thing that any parent would do if their child had a rare or undiagnosed condition. 'I *would* be asking for a second opinion. Of course I'd be pushing for educational support for my child if that was appropriate. If I thought I'd been given a duff diagnosis, I would be questioning it. I absolutely would be that pushy parent,' she says.

'If you think about it from the mindset of a parent in that position, it's exactly what you would do to try and help your child, but then you've ticked all the boxes for FII. You're completely damned whatever you do as a mum – and it is normally mums,' Emma adds. 'I'd love to know if dads are less likely to be accused. I don't think anyone's ever looked into it, and unfortunately it is still quite rare for dads to bring their kid to an appointment.'

*

Of course, none of this is to say that mothers always know best, any more than doctors do. But if both parties have the child's best interests at heart, surely the relationship should be one of collaboration, rather than conflict or even competition?

'You can probably split sick children into two types. There's those who had been previously fit and well, who then have a problem – a chest infection, a broken arm or something – and there you're just going to have to take the parent's word for what's going on. You've also got chronically unwell children, where you've got a lot of information on file, but the parent is an evolving advocate for that child, who undoubtedly understands their child's illness better than you do at that particular point,' explains Dr Keir Shiels.

'You can also divide parents into those who are inexperienced and unsupported, and those who are more experienced,' he adds. Parents without a supportive family network might be very worried about relatively minor things, Keir explains, because they haven't got people around them to say, 'Don't worry, you used to do that.' More experienced parents, on the other hand, may present a bit later, or only with more significant concerns.

The other notable gender gap Keir sees, particularly working in a multicultural area of London, is around language barriers. 'We see families where the mother is the primary carer for the child but has very little spoken English, so is unable to communicate what their problems and concerns are. Particularly during the pandemic, where we've only been allowed to see one parent with their child, we've had to choose between the mother, who knows what's wrong but can't tell us, or the father, who typically can speak English but doesn't know anything about what's wrong,' he explains.

Keir believes part of the problem, particularly for new, inexperienced mothers, is that medicine is not good enough at informing women of what is 'normal' and to be expected when you have a baby: 'We don't talk enough about the fact that breastfeeding is difficult or that every baby on the planet gets jaundice. We don't talk about the fact that interpreting your baby's crying or dealing with reflux is a hard thing.'

As a result, he adds, for every mother like Lui, who was right to be very worried and tenacious, there are probably 99 examples of mothers who simply needed some empathy, compassion and reassurance. Likewise, Keir says, for every 10 mothers who come into a consultation with research printed out from Dr Google, five will have got it right, four will have got it very wrong and one will just be throwing out darts, desperately trying to find out what's wrong.

'You see the whole range of parents, from the ones who actively make decisions that will harm their child, through to parents who are very, very anxious about totally normal things. There's a huge range of different ways in which people interpret facts and risks, so it's hard; it's really tough,' he says.

'The necessity of infallibility is the hardest thing; you're not allowed to make a mistake as a doctor. You're not allowed to be that GP who got it wrong. Having seen 25 babies with exactly the same thing, all of whom got better, you can't get the 26th one wrong, because that makes you unprofessional and seem like a moron. That mum is never going to go back to that GP and yet the other 25 would trust him or her implicitly.'

When it comes to more experienced mothers, however, particularly those with chronically ill children, Keir says, 'Woe betide any paediatrician who doesn't listen to a mother's instinct. You have to listen to the parent and work together.' With poorly understood conditions like ME, he adds, the emergence of Long Covid has demonstrated how evidence changes and evolves; that nothing in medical science is certain. But, he says, 'Being radical in medicine is considered a very dangerous thing. It's a lot easier to believe everything we've been taught than to reassess it. In cases where there's uncertainty, honesty and teamwork are the only solution.'

This, too, is not without its challenges. 'There are times when the parent's insight or agenda is distinct from your understanding of the disease. Those are very difficult conversations, because you're going on a journey with somebody where your two interpretations of the same piece of information are different. In some cases, the parent is wrong. In others, it might be more up for debate. There are lots of decisions to be made, but ultimately it's their call as long as it's in their child's best interests,' he explains.

*

Steph Nimmo is the author of *Was This in the Plan?*, and has explored the complexities of this relationship from the other side of the fence. Her daughter Daisy, the youngest of Steph's four children, was born in 2004 with the rare, life-limiting genetic disease Costello Syndrome, plunging Steph into an unfamiliar medical world. Daisy was in and out of Great Ormond Street Hospital throughout her short life, before dying in early 2017, at the age of 12.

In many respects, Steph says, her experiences with Daisy's doctors and nurses were very positive. 'With Daisy's first consultant I just felt like I was talking to another mum. She sat me down, we had a cup of coffee away from the ward and she was very open with me. Having someone like that who I could turn to made a massive difference,' she says.

During the early years, though, Steph recalls feeling lost and disempowered. 'It was like people were speaking a different language and assuming I would understand, or talking at me instead of to me,' she tells me – and her research has confirmed she's not the only mother to feel this way. 'Whatever background you come from, and no matter how experienced you are, when you're parenting a child like Daisy there are those feelings of total, utter disempowerment and not being listened to,' Steph says.

'I've interviewed a former palliative care nurse who now has a terminally ill child and she, despite all her professional experience, still was not taken seriously, still had to fight, still beats herself up for not pushing when it turned out her instinct was right.'

For Steph, though, the biggest turning point was realising, quite early on, that medicine didn't have all the answers. 'I just didn't know how the system worked. I assumed that once Daisy was transferred to Great Ormond Street it would be okay and everyone would know what was going on, but they didn't,' she says. As the parent of a child with a complex, poorly understood disease, Steph was stunned to realise how much academic guesswork was going to be involved in Daisy's care. 'It was almost exactly the same feeling as the moment when you realise, as a child, that your parents are actually fallible,' she says.

'In some ways that became quite empowering for me, because it shifted the whole power dynamic. I realised my child really needed me to know what the hell was going on. The doctors didn't have all the answers, and I needed to work collaboratively with healthcare staff and find out who was going to help me. I saw my role as trying to give them information on what I knew about Daisy's rare disease.'

Up until this point, Steph had been a successful, professional working woman, heading up a department as a senior manager – a role she gave up in order to care for Daisy. From all her conversations with other parents, Steph believes there is a huge gender bias in the assumption that women will assume the role of carer. 'I automatically thought, "I'll give up my job and care for Daisy." Looking back, I'm like, what the hell? I was the major wage earner, why was I giving up my job? But at the same time, I couldn't *not* look after Daisy, so I was my own worst enemy too,' she says.

While to some extent this professional experience gave her the confidence and authority to advocate successfully on behalf of her child, it still came as a huge cultural shift to find herself reduced to the role of full-time mother. Writing for the *BMJ* in 2019, Steph describes her frustration at continuously being addressed as 'Mum' by members of Daisy's healthcare team, which led to the hashtag #DontCallMeMum. 'I felt so dehumanised and depersonalised by just being seen as "Daisy's mum". Being called "Mum" made me feel like I'd lost myself. I found that I really had to earn the right for my knowledge and expertise to be taken seriously – they had to get to know me,' Steph tells me. 'Equally, I wanted them to get to know Daisy as a little girl, not just an "interesting case".'

Looking back on the dynamic her late husband Andy had with hospital staff, Steph also believes the gendered differences work both ways. 'The way he interacted with healthcare professionals was sometimes not so conducive to collaboration, like he'd get really cross if mistakes were made. But there was also a difference in the way the mostly female healthcare staff responded to him. It's difficult to put my finger on it, but I always felt that the nurses wanted to help the dads, whereas the mums [were expected to] just get on with it,' she says.

Steph recalls one night in particular, at gone midnight, when she was concerned that Daisy's intravenous medications, which she needed at regular intervals throughout the day, had not been administered. 'I told the nurse that Daisy needed to sleep, I needed to sleep – I was exhausted – and she just said, "That's what being a parent is all about." I was so furious I nearly hit her, because I knew she would never have said that to my husband.' As she says it, I'm immediately reminded of Clare Murphy's words, at the start of this chapter. As Clare so rightly observes, maternal self-sacrifice is simply what's expected of mothers – whether that means sacrificing their career, their identity or even just their sleep.

How then can healthcare professionals bridge this gap and collaborate better with the mothers of sick – diagnosed or otherwise – children? For Steph it's always boiled down to three things: 'Firstly, remember that the parent carers – the women who live this 24/7 – deserve a seat at the table because they bring a view of the situation that the healthcare professionals will never have,' she says.

Secondly, Steph adds, 'It's okay to say you don't know. I'd be more worried if my daughter had tonsillitis and the doctor didn't know what to do. But when you're at the edge of medical science, saying we need to work together becomes a lot more empowering than being given false hope.' Finally, she says, 'Take off the metaphorical white coat and have some empathy. How would you feel if it was your child? In many ways I've found that doctors hide behind all the technical speak, but they're actually scared. What do I say? How do I have this difficult conversation? It's okay just to feel it.'

This, she acknowledges, is not a straightforward ask, particularly in busy, under-resourced wards where every mother wants their child to be the number-one priority. Can doctors really be expected to show empathy under such intense pressure or to allow themselves to feel emotionally attached to seriously unwell, life-limited children? 'I don't know how they protect themselves emotionally and psychologically from all the things they must see,' Steph admits.

'I do see a lot of burnout among healthcare professionals. They're parents themselves, they may have their own health issues, and the good ones definitely don't do it for the money! The dehumanisation does work both ways; there is a dehumanisation of healthcare professionals by patients, which really does need to change as well. We're all human.'

Again, as we've seen so often already, a lot of the difficulties come back to doctors simply not having the time to listen. 'In GP surgeries you've basically got about eight minutes. In emergency medicine you've technically got as long as you want, in the sense that the only patient you're dealing with is the emergency in the room, but you're aware that you've got a queue of other emergencies behind you that also need to be dealt with. In clinic you've also got a waiting room outside,' Keir explains.

'Under that time pressure, you've got to foster an environment in which people who've never met you before can tell you their secrets. That takes time and it takes trust. Everyone brings their own insights and their own fears into the consultation room, and unpicking the psychology of why a mum or dad is worried is a huge challenge.'

Empathy with the patient, he says, is much easier in many ways. 'It's much easier to be empathetic when your patient is six because, however minor an issue you're dealing with, it's still the worst thing that's ever happened to that six-year-old.' That said, there are still tragedies that affect him, although for the most part he tries to contextualise these and work out what a good outcome would look like. 'I have seen enough really, really happy disabled children now, for example, that when I break the news to people that their child is going to be disabled, I can give some positive outlook,' he says.

'Sometimes, though, bad stuff just happens for no reason. I don't want that sort of stuff to stop affecting me; the day that I'm unaffected by it is the day I'm walking out of medicine. If you can't cry with somebody then there is a big problem about your emotional understanding of the situation. You need to be able to hold somebody and be reassuring. If you can give both the patient and their parent a bit of perspective, that does help.'

YOUR PAEDIATRIC HEALTH TOOLKIT

Motherhood is hard, and I suspect there's no amount of tips and advice that will change that. They say it takes a village to raise a child, but being a mum can be incredibly lonely, particularly if you don't have your own or your partner's mum to call on for support and guidance. Whatever your starting point, build yourself that village, be it via online support groups, local parenting groups and other mum friends, or apps like Peanut. This will give you a sounding board against which to gauge how normal or otherwise your child's symptoms are and whether or not you should be concerned. If in doubt, though, trust your instinct and get them checked out.

If your child has ongoing, unexplained symptoms that you feel are not being taken seriously, Eos Advocacy, a specialist support service for families, recommends documenting everything carefully. 'Keep a diary of symptoms, alongside records of when third parties, such as in education and healthcare, have witnessed them. Keep records of calls and emails, and follow up by email on any symptoms occurring in an education setting that you are informed of verbally,' says Emma Louise, director of Eos Advocacy.

'Whilst anxieties may naturally occur, it is important that these are not projected onto the child. They should be supported to live as best possible in line with their peers, with reasonable adjustments in place,' she adds. 'Unfortunately advocating for your child or being knowledgeable about a condition can be seen as a red flag, but parents should absolutely uphold their child's best interests to avoid detrimental effects on the child's emotional and physical wellbeing.'

Above all, whatever you and your child are going through, remember to look after yourself as well, and reach out to relevant charities or organisations for emotional and moral support.

Resources

- Bright Futures UK – brightfuturesuk.org
- Carers UK – carersuk.org
- Eos Advocacy – eosadvocacy.co.uk
- Medical Mediation Foundation – medicalmediation .org.uk
- Not Fine In School – notfineinschool.co.uk
- Rainbow Trust – rainbowtrust.org.uk
- Sick Children's Trust – sickchildrenstrust.org
- Special Needs Jungle – specialneedsjungle.com
- Sunshine Support – sunshine-support.org
- Together For Short Lives – togetherforshortlives.org.uk
- Was This In The Plan? – wasthisintheplan.co.uk/@ StephNimmo
- Well Child – wellchild.org.uk

10

'Menopausal crones': When sexism and ageism collide

Much like menstruation, the menopause has been having a bit of a moment in recent years – thanks, in no small part, to the tireless efforts of patient advocates speaking out. A flurry of books, articles, blogs, podcasts and documentaries have begun to bring the menopause out of the shadows, with public figures like Davina McCall, Jenny Eclair, Liz Earle and Meg Matthews shining a light on what has been, perhaps, the ultimate taboo in women's health.

The menopause – officially diagnosed after 12 months without menstrual periods – will affect half the population at some point in their lives. Yet it's a subject on which many of us, and our doctors, remain woefully misinformed and underprepared. A 2020 survey conducted by the Female Founders Fund revealed that just 36% of the 250 respondents felt 'moderately or very prepared' for menopause, and 32% felt their doctors were not knowledgeable or confident discussing the subject.

A larger scale survey, conducted by Nuffield Health, found that one in four women experiencing menopause symptoms were 'concerned about their ability to cope with life' with 62% reporting symptoms that resulted in changes to their behaviour or which had a detrimental effect on their lives. Meanwhile, 67% said there was a general lack of support or advice for those going through the menopause and one in 10 had considered leaving their jobs as a result. Indeed, 2021 research by Newson Health showed that roughly one in five women in perimenopause reduce their hours or don't go for promotions they would otherwise have considered, while 12% actually do resign.

The taboos surrounding menopause are hardly surprising. As we know, virtually all health issues that primarily affect women are poorly understood and under-prioritised. Much like with periods, difficult menopause symptoms are easily dismissed as 'normal', 'natural', 'part of being a woman' and something we 'just have to put up with.' With menopause, though, that sexism also collides quite spectacularly with a broader societal ageism that says older women – those past their sexually attractive, baby-making prime – simply aren't that important anymore. In the media and in the workplace, these women are seen as past it, 'dried up', and gradually become more and more invisible as they age.

In healthcare, you see this particularly in attitudes towards post-menopausal sexual pain and dysfunction. Vaginal atrophy, which affects as many as one in three women in menopause, is a drying and thinning of the vaginal tissue, caused by depleted oestrogen levels. It can lead to pain, itching and discomfort, as well as frequent UTIs, vaginal bleeding and painful sex. Simple and effective treatments for vaginal atrophy include local oestrogen – applied to the vagina as a cream, pessary or ring – as well as over-the-counter moisturisers and lubricants. Yet, as Jane Lewis, author of *Me & My Menopausal Vagina*, tells me, 'far too many' women affected by vaginal atrophy are 'dismissed and ridiculed'.

This isn't just frustrating; it also has a serious impact on relationships. According to research carried out for the *Independent* in 2021, 65% of women aged 40 and over believe being menopausal has impacted their marriage. Almost half the 534 women surveyed said they had stopped having sex during the menopause and a similar number believed 'their relationship could have been rescued if the NHS had better help for those struggling with symptoms.'

There's an unspoken belief, it seems, that women above a certain age are too old, too sexually unappealing for sex anyway – and certainly too old to want or expect to enjoy it. Instead, women are told they should simply tolerate their discomfort, self-medicate with alcohol, or even find other ways to pleasure their husbands – because that, of course, is the main thing. 'Would a GP's response be the same if a man got his penis out, his GP could see it was sore, splitting and itchy, and he said that every time he had sex he would get a UTI?' Jane asks. 'I am pretty certain it would not.'

Similarly, the changes typically occurring for women during this time in their life mean cognitive and mental health symptoms of menopause are often misdiagnosed as depression, stress or anxiety. Mental health issues affect as many as 90% of women during menopause and women aged 45–64 have the highest female suicide rate in England and Wales. Too often, though, these struggles are dismissively attributed to mid-life challenges like children leaving home, caring for ageing parents, or going through career or relationship changes. Although NICE guidelines are clear that antidepressants should not generally be used as a first-line treatment for menopausal mood changes, many GPs continue to inappropriately prescribe antidepressants rather than looking at hormonal causes and treatments.

Katie Taylor spent four years of her mid-40s being 'made to feel like I was losing my mind'. As well as low mood and anxiety, Katie struggled with forgetfulness and cognitive difficulties known as 'brain fog', which were so bad she became convinced she was suffering from early onset dementia. The first GP she saw diagnosed depression and prescribed antidepressants. The next said it was stress from juggling too much and suggested she give up work – which she did.

When her periods also became very heavy, making Katie anaemic, it was her father – a breast cancer surgeon – who suggested the cause might be hormonal. Sure enough, a blood test and a consultation with a gynaecologist confirmed Katie was in perimenopause. 'She explained that my oestrogen levels were on the floor and were the entire reason I was feeling all these things. She reassured me that nothing was wrong with me, suggested I have a coil fitted to stop the bleeding, and told me I'd feel like a new woman after a month on hormone replacement therapy (HRT).'

Four weeks later, Katie adds, 'My mood had lifted significantly, my energy levels had peaked, my memory returned, I could think clearly and make normal decisions, the anxiety and palpitations stopped, and I suddenly realised I was happy and really enjoying my life again.' In relief, she founded the Latte Lounge, a Facebook support group and website for women over 40, which now has more than 20,000 members.

Many of these, she discovered, had been through similar experiences, feeling alone, lost and confused in the face of symptoms they didn't understand and GPs who'd failed to make the link to menopause. According to a survey by menopause specialist Newson Health, 7% of menopausal women visit their GP more than 10 times and 44% wait at least a year before receiving adequate help or advice. Even for patients who make the connection themselves, the general lack of awareness and training among GPs may leave them dismissed, denied treatment or even told they're 'too young' for the menopause.

However, the reality, as many people who experience it are shocked to discover, is that menopause symptoms can begin much earlier than we've been led to believe. While most women and people who menstruate will stop having periods naturally between 45 and 55 years of age – with 51 the average – symptoms typically begin during your 40s. This transition period, when oestrogen levels begin to decline, is known as perimenopause and can start months or years before your periods actually stop.

For others, an early menopause may be brought on by premature ovarian insufficiency (POI, which affects around

1% of women under 40), by surgical removal of the ovaries (an oophorectomy) or certain medical treatments. With our population living longer, many of us will therefore spend half our lives in a state of perimenopause or post-menopause and we deserve for that second half to be just as happy, fulfilling and, yes, even sexually satisfying as the first.

The catalogue of potential menopause symptoms includes hot flushes, night sweats, vaginal atrophy, brain fog, reduced libido, menstrual cycle changes, depression and anxiety, as well as longer term risks associated with reduced oestrogen, like osteoporosis and cardiovascular disease. It's also worth noting that, just as we've seen with both period symptoms and contraceptive side-effects, different people experience hormonal changes differently – and we still don't fully understand why. While one woman may breeze through the menopause, others suffer far more severely and in very different ways.

'Natural' and 'normal' as all these symptoms may be, that doesn't mean anyone should be expected to put up with them, particularly if they're having a debilitating impact on their everyday life. Such suffering is not simply an inconvenient but unavoidable part of living with ageing ovaries and, crucially, we have safe and effective treatment options with which to do something about it.

This in itself has been problematic, with flawed studies and scaremongering media coverage during the early 2000s generating widespread concern about the risks associated with HRT, the main treatment recommended for menopausal symptoms. Breast cancer scares in particular saw women come off HRT and doctors stop prescribing it en masse two decades ago. However, recent evidence shows that the risk of breast cancer was overstated. Certainly for anyone already living with, or at high risk of, hormonally driven conditions – including oestrogen-sensitive forms of breast cancer – HRT is likely not to be recommended, and doctors should work with patients to explore alternative solutions. For the majority of people though, the benefits of taking HRT outweigh the risks. Despite this, many patients and GPs alike continue to fear using or prescribing it.

As the name suggests, HRT works by replacing the natural hormones that are in decline – typically oestrogen. This is given in combination with progestogen to anyone who still has their uterus, as oestrogen alone slightly increases the risk of womb cancer. Testosterone cream may also be prescribed by menopause specialists to help with reduced libido. However, as testosterone is not currently licensed for use by women in the UK, many non-specialists are reluctant to prescribe it.

Newer forms of HRT are plant-based (unlike the more off-putting older forms, derived from equine urine) and 'body identical', meaning they more closely mimic your body's natural oestrogen. They come in various forms and combinations, including patches, gels and sprays that are applied to the skin and are safer for those at higher risk of blood clots. Like hormonal contraceptives, it can take some trial and error to find the right type and dose of HRT for each individual patient's needs, and this again is where the lack of specialist knowledge in primary care can become a real barrier to accessing the best possible care.

Dr Nighat Arif is one of the brilliant NHS GPs who's trying to change all that from the inside out. 'There is a big problem with misogyny within healthcare. A woman is only seen as fit for purpose when she's reproducing; when she's stopped reproducing, when she's menopausal, well that's just "normal". Anything in medicine that's seen as "normal" is going to be under-researched because it's not a priority,' she says.

'We've seen a lot of misinformation about HRT, which came out of flawed studies, and menopause care has never been a mandatory part of medical education for healthcare professionals,' Nighat adds. 'We don't teach doctors about menopause and how to identify the seemingly hotchpotch symptoms or the options for HRT. If you're a GP you can do an optional e-module, which is very basic and hasn't really been updated, or if you have a really keen interest in menopause you can go to the British Menopause

Society and get an accreditation certificate. That's an interesting course, but it's quite expensive and you have to spend your own time and money on it; it's not covered by the NHS,' she explains.

In an ideal world, Nighat adds, all healthcare professionals should know about menopause, not just GPs. If you're working in orthopaedics, for example, you may be performing hip replacements on post-menopausal women with osteoporosis. Those working in geriatrics, on the other hand, may encounter women with pain and discomfort caused by vaginal atrophy. Yet currently only the most interested and proactive doctors will have sought out training on an issue that affects half their patients who are middle-aged or beyond. When you combine the ongoing fear of HRT with this broader lack of understanding, knowledge and concern about the menopause, it's easy to see how those going through 'the change' are so often left to suffer in silence.

✶

Since 2018, Diane Danzebrink has been the face of a patient-led menopause movement, but just six years earlier she entered the menopause herself, utterly clueless about what awaited her. Diane was in her mid-40s at the time, and had undergone a total hysterectomy and oophorectomy after cysts were discovered on both her ovaries.

'My mother had ovarian cancer in her 40s and doctors suspected I also had ovarian cancer, so I was booked in for surgery relatively quickly,' she explains. 'I knew that once my ovaries were gone, I'd be in the menopause, but I thought that would just mean no more periods and probably hot flushes. That's all I knew. Doctors repeated to me several times that I would lose my fertility, but I'd already made a considered decision not to have children. Apart from that, there was no focus on the aftermath.'

After her surgery, Diane was discharged and went home to recover in front of the London 2012 Olympics. She was given no information about surgical menopause, despite the fact this abrupt loss of oestrogen can result in more severe symptoms than going through perimenopause naturally.

When her histology report came back, Diane was relieved to learn that her ovaries were not cancerous. The surgery had, however, found and relieved her of extensive undiagnosed endometriosis, adenomyosis and a large fibroid, which finally explained the painful and heavy periods that doctors had fobbed her off about for years previously. 'I just thought all I want to do now is crack on and get well again, get on with my life,' Diane says. 'I'd already heard all the scary stuff about HRT from 20 years previously and decided I didn't want that; I'd just deal with menopause the natural way.'

At first, Diane says, everything was fine apart from a few hot flushes. Within a few months, though, her mental health had taken a dramatic turn for the worse. 'I started to become increasingly anxious and overwhelmed. The world started to feel like a very dark and scary place. I'd regularly wake up with my heart racing, feeling as though there was somebody sitting on my chest, and have to wake my husband in a panic,' she recalls.

'It became a downward spiral to the point where I wouldn't leave the house. I was no longer able to work. I wouldn't answer the telephone or even open a letter, because I had become so irrationally fearful of what might be in it. The only people I would see were my husband and my mum. My husband got so worried about me that he had to get my mum to come and stay with us so he could carry on going out to work. I genuinely thought I was going mad,' Diane adds.

The breaking point came after she spent an entire day plucking up the courage to call her local surgery and ask if there was a menopause support service she could speak to. 'The woman I spoke to was lovely, but she just said, "I'm sorry my dear, there's no such thing." I literally fell into the sofa and sobbed and sobbed and sobbed. I was completely inconsolable, because that had felt like my last option. I just became this non-functioning husk of a person,' she says.

It wasn't until later, after Diane had come perilously close to taking her own life, that she finally saw a GP who really took the time to explain the hormonal changes she was going through and provide good, evidence-based information about HRT. 'It was an enormous relief to go on HRT patches and feel the clouds start to lift a little bit. But then I got angry, because it made me wonder how many people have not been fortunate enough to have the amazing family support that I had, who never got the right advice and support,' she says.

'Having done the work I do now, I know for a fact there are an awful lot of them, but back then it just made me wonder. I'd been told there was no national menopause support service and none of the clinicians I'd seen previously – including the surgeon who took my ovaries away – had ever told me what the effects could be. It wasn't until the point of crisis that I was fortunate enough to be put in front of someone who did understand it. I just thought no, this can't go on, I'm going to make damn sure I do something to change this,' Diane adds.

In 2015, after attending nurse training in menopause, Diane used her background in counselling and coaching to launch Menopause Support, providing one-to-one support as well as factual, evidence-based information for other people going through the menopause. Two years later, after also launching a Facebook support group that now has more than 25,000 members, Diane decided she needed to do more. 'I was sat one night at my computer and got another desperate email from a woman, and I just thought, this is ridiculous; we can't go on like this. I decided we needed a national campaign,' she explains.

That campaign was #MakeMenopauseMatter and the petition Diane set up that evening has at the time of writing attracted more than 165,000 signatures. Buoyed by the broader movement for menstrual health education, within a year of launching her campaign Diane had succeeded in getting menopause education added to the school curriculum in England, as part of mandatory lessons on sex, relationships and health. These have been in place since September 2021, but, Diane says, there's still an 'overwhelming need' for more to be done.

The final two demands of #MakeMenopauseMatter are guidance and support in every workplace, to help keep menopausal employees in their careers and, most crucially, mandatory menopause education for all GPs. Ultimately, like Nighat, Diane tells me she'd like to see this put in place for all healthcare professionals, but GPs are an essential first step. In their primary care role, as we've seen elsewhere, GPs so often act as the gatekeepers between patients and specialist support, and Diane says there are plenty of recurring themes that come up time and again in the issues she hears about daily.

'If somebody is under 50, particularly if they're under 45, they may be told they're too young for menopause. Or it can't be menopause, because you're still having periods. There's a complete lack of recognition of premature ovarian insufficiency (early menopause) and a lot of fear and misinformation about HRT, like you can't have HRT until your periods have stopped – which just isn't true,' she explains.

'There's also still a lack of recognition of the plethora of menopause symptoms. So many healthcare professionals don't recognise how many symptoms there are, particularly psychological ones, so these are very often explained away. I really don't think this should be a patient vs doctor conversation, but I'm sad to say I do also still hear from women who've been laughed at, or had doctors raise their voice in frustration, and that's not acceptable.'

Although patients can ask their GP to refer them to a specialist menopause clinic, there isn't always one available locally, and the waiting lists for these services are typically very long – leaving many people with limited alternatives. As a result, Diane adds, another, often hidden issue is the debt some women get into in pursuit of a diagnosis and treatment.

'So many women who've had several appointments and are not being correctly diagnosed, not being heard, or have been refused the treatment they'd like to try, are being forced down the private route. That's absolutely fine if you're fortunate enough to be able to afford that, but we're hearing from women who've put it on a credit card, or even applied for a credit card to be able to do it. Some have taken loans from family members or dipped into small savings pots that they'd put aside for something else,' she explains.

It's worth noting that, exactly as we've seen with menstruation, the rise in patient conversations about the menopause has ushered in huge commercial interest in the field. Recent years have seen an explosion of private menopause care and slick new menopause-friendly brands, offering everything from private prescriptions to herbal remedies, cosmetics, lotions and potions, some more reputable – and more expensive – than others. In 2021, research from Diane's Menopause Support network found that 48% of more than 600 women surveyed had been left with no option but to seek private menopause care, with some of them going thousands of pounds into debt.

In 2021 the Ginsburg Women's Health Board, along with other campaigners, launched a campaign to make HRT prescriptions free in England, as they already are in Scotland and Wales. The compromise announced by then health secretary Sajid Javid was an annual prepayment scheme, allowing patients to pay a single annual prescription fee of £18.70 for their HRT, saving them up to £205 a year. This is due to be introduced in April 2023 but, of course, is only of any help if your GP will agree to prescribe HRT in the first place. 'There's enormous demand and it really puts vulnerable women in a difficult position. If you can't get the treatment you need from your GP, where do you go? You either go without or you dip back into a non-existent pot and then you're trapped,' Diane says. 'We are hearing of more doctors who have done some training and are more up to date, but we need that across the board. There's absolutely no reason why it should be a lottery.'

Reduced price prescriptions are also not much use if you can't get hold of the treatment you need. Shortages of certain HRT products were reported across the UK in 2019 and again in 2022, with the reasons given ranging from supply chain issues to a massive increase in demand. In 2022 the government launched an HRT Taskforce and introduced limits on some products in an effort to relieve issues and support the supply chain. Yet the campaigners I spoke to, quite fairly, wanted to know why this hadn't been prioritised three years earlier, to prevent shortages like the ones seen in 2019 from happening again.

There's also a vitally important conversation to be had about non-hormonal solutions to menopause symptoms – both to complement HRT and as stand-alone treatments in their own right for anyone who can't, or doesn't want to, use hormone replacement therapy. For some in this group, the menopause movement's increasing focus on HRT advocacy has understandably felt alienating. When it comes to supporting everyone to find their own best way through the menopause, plenty of other options – including pharmaceuticals, alternative therapies, nutrition and weight-bearing exercise – also have a role to play.

✶

Diane and her campaign have been instrumental in opening up the menopause conversation to a much broader audience. For Dr Nighat Arif, it's now vital to ensure all patients can benefit from this movement, including those from ethnic minority backgrounds. 'I'm a practising Muslim and started my GP work in a predominantly Pakistani community, where women's health is still a massive taboo,' she says. 'If you've got painful periods or severe hot flushes, you grin and bear it, or you use faith as a coping strategy. Both of these limit women from going out and seeking appropriate help from their doctors.'

But cultural taboos are not the only barrier. Non-white representation is woeful, both in menopause research and in the public conversation. The limited research we do have, Nighat tells me, suggests that menopausal women from ethnic minority communities are more likely than white women to leave the workforce, leaving them financially vulnerable. We also know these patient groups have a higher risk of heart disease, but there's little public recognition of the impact menopause can have on cardiovascular health.

'When you're under-researching these communities and you're not making the health benefits of HRT known to them, preventative healthcare can't happen,' Nighat says. 'We're picking up these patients too late. You could avoid vaginal atrophy if you give someone oestrogen earlier. Or you could prevent heart disease or osteoporosis. That's what really upsets me, because preventative medicine is what we should be practising; it's cheaper for the NHS and it's better for the patients.'

Equally, she adds, both data and her own experience indicate that ethnic minority women are less likely to complain of the classic well-known menopause symptoms like hot flushes, night sweats and irritability, but may report aches and pains, stiffness, fatigue, headaches, itchy skin or eyes, or blurred vision. This highlights again how important it is for doctors to understand the huge range of possible symptoms and how they may affect different patient groups differently. It's also, Nighat feels, why it's so important for her to be visibly outspoken about these issues as a Muslim woman in a hijab – to give a voice and representation to women who so rarely see themselves represented in this space.

Likewise, both research and representation are virtually non-existent when it comes to menopause in the LGBTQ+ community. 'The literature [on menopause] focuses almost completely on heterosexual experiences and assumes that only women experience menopause,' writes psychotherapist Tania Glyde in their research exploring how therapists can best support queer menopausal clients, which was published in 2021. 'Aside from some studies which include lesbian experience, there is almost no peer-reviewed literature about queer experience of menopause.'

Through their interviews with 12 LGBTQ+ participants Tania's research lays bare a catalogue of negative experiences with GPs. These participants included cis bisexual, asexual and queer women, as well as trans, non-binary and genderqueer people. While seeking medical care during menopause, many of these patients faced the same dearth of knowledge, information and understanding as cis straight women like Diane, but combined with the ignorance, biases and inappropriate treatment we've seen LGBTQ+ patients encounter elsewhere in medicine.

Perhaps most shocking is the 'humiliating' interrogation of genderqueer lesbian patient Robin, who describes being aggressively questioned about their genitalia, their gender and gender-affirming treatments. Others spoke about having to educate their GP about their gender and sexuality, seeing multiple different doctors before finding one who was helpful, and having to do their own research in order to be their 'own doctor'.

Another alarming theme, which Tania says was echoed in several interviews, is the non-consensual writing of prescriptions, including for antidepressants. 'When they went to their GP to talk about menopause, pansexual non-binary patient Bret was told they should be on antidepressants. Bret disagreed, saying they did not want to lose their libido (for them a vital part of their queer identity). The GP wrote the prescription anyway. When menopause comes into the frame, it feels like a licence to infantilise patients,' they write.

'Really, inclusion and awareness need to be built in from the ground up, and all staff need to be trained, not just GPs. Doctors need to know the impact on a patient of having to explain their sexuality and/or gender, and sometimes having to justify it. But it starts before they get into the clinic – reception staff need to be trained about pronouns and changes of name and not, as in some cases, discount the patient's needs or even laugh at them. Unfortunately, this is still happening,' Tania tells me.

For trans men and trans masculine people in particular, there's also a real issue with the lack of medical knowledge and understanding about both surgical menopause (for those who undergo a hysterectomy and oophorectomy) and the impact of testosterone treatment. 'Some practitioners have this knowledge, but it doesn't yet seem to be joined up. I'm starting to get more enquiries about this and would like to find knowledgeable people to refer clients to, but currently there just isn't enough easily accessible information out there,' they add.

As a way of beginning to bridge this information gap, Tania launched Queer Menopause, an online resource and blog to continue exploring LGBTQ+ experiences of menopause that have long been invisible. 'There was nothing else like it and I wanted somewhere to put my research and anything else I could find,' they say. 'I've seen a lot of demand for this conversation – both from people who hadn't realised the LGBTQIA+ experience might be different from a straight cis woman's, and from LGBTQIA+ people who had been sitting in silence wondering what was going on with them and not realising there were others experiencing the same thing.'

Fashion designer Karen Arthur tells me she was similarly frustrated by the absence of Black women's voices from the menopause conversation. In the wake of George Floyd's murder she founded Menopause Whilst Black, a podcast and Instagram account where she interviews Black women about their experiences. 'I'd been having these conversations about menopause with some of my friends around my kitchen table for the previous two years, but I realised we needed more; we needed a platform for Black British women. It was one of those things where I'd been looking around thinking, "Someone else will do that," and then it dawned on me, "Oh God, it's going to be me, isn't it?" But I couldn't not speak; I didn't have a choice,' she tells me.

Karen was 'completely and utterly unprepared' for the menopause. 'I just thought I was dying, I couldn't cope with it,' she recalls. 'I was 51 when I realised I was going through the menopause and first heard the term perimenopause.' While

Karen did experience physical symptoms like tingly legs and hot flushes – which she initially assumed was just a fault with her new boiler – it was her mental health that took the biggest hit. Eight months after her final period, Karen was signed off work with depression and anxiety. 'All my knowledge and understanding of my perimenopausal experience is more recent and retrospective,' she adds.

During the 'Blackout' summer of 2020, while Black Lives Matter demonstrations took place across the globe, Karen was researching. 'I found out from the (US-based) Study of Women's Health Across the Nation (SWAN) report that Black women are more likely to start menopause up to two years earlier than their white counterparts, and we're also more likely to suffer from hot flushes more severely.

'I kept thinking, "How the f*ck is this not common knowledge and why are Black women not being told this so they can prepare?" I didn't understand how we were coping with that, while also coping with seeing people who look like us or our families being murdered, and recognising that racism is very much alive and kicking,' she explains. 'I started asking questions, launched a survey, then I started the Instagram account and the podcast. It's been phenomenal to get more Black women talking about the menopause and people really seem to get it.'

Around the same time, Nina Kuypers was having similar conversations on Twitter and Facebook, and launched Black Women in Menopause – a platform which, like Karen's, provides a space for Black women to access information and support for their experiences, as well as educational events. Now three years post-menopause, changes to Nina's hair and skin have been among the biggest impacts she's experienced since first entering perimenopause in her mid-40s. But even as businesses rush to cash in on the growing menopause conversation, products designed for Black skin and hair are notably absent from the influx of new brands targeting midlife women in high street pharmacies.

Since launching Menopause Whilst Black, Karen says two of the biggest themes to come out of her interviews have been a culture of 'soldiering on', and a deep-rooted yet understandable mistrust of doctors and medicine. 'There's a recognition of the racism behind how modern medicine came to be, like the legacy of Dr Marion Sims, and a feeling of not being listened to by doctors, and not trusting them or trusting medication like HRT,' Karen says.

'But there's also this attitude that "Well, my mother soldiered on, so I'm going to soldier on." There's something about our culture, both African and Caribbean, around being the strong Black woman, which includes not using drugs to help you. I was dead set against HRT as well until a year ago. It was appearing on the *Sex, Myths and the Menopause* documentary with Davina [McCall] that really opened my eyes,' she adds.

The big question, of course, is how can the healthcare profession even begin to start tackling this mistrust? 'I don't know. But I do know that outwards, obvious anti-racism training would be a good start and true investment in diversity,' Karen says. 'Tackling racism is huge. It will involve making a lot of people very uncomfortable and removing people from positions of power who've been there for years. It has to come from the top down and there has to be a global conversation about menopause that includes Black women, Asian women, LGBTQ+ people, all the people who are going to transition through menopause, which also includes the men in their lives.'

*

It's also vital that these conversations extend beyond those in their 40s and 50s, recognising the risks and gender health gaps that exist well into old age. Women, for example, outnumber men two to one when it comes to dementia diagnoses and it's only really in the last few years that science has begun to scratch the surface of understanding why.

The factors behind the dementia gap are complex and still not well understood. It may in part be down to the fact that dementia risk increases with age and women typically live longer than men. However, scientists believe there are also biological factors at play – and the role of hormones could be a significant one. Research shows that oestrogen has a protective effect on the brain, which, according to the Alzheimer's Society, could explain why the sudden drop in women's oestrogen levels following the menopause seems to make them more vulnerable to Alzheimer's and other forms of dementia.

It could also help to explain the forgetfulness and 'brain fog' that many women, like Katie, experience around perimenopause. While these cognitive difficulties are usually temporary, the *New York Times Magazine* reports that they are more likely to have a lasting impact on low-income women of colour. This, according to Professor Pauline Maki, is 'probably because those women have higher rates of stress, disrupted sleep and other mental health burdens that make the brain more vulnerable.'

There are also question marks around the role of HRT in preventing dementia, with research so far showing conflicting results. While some studies suggest HRT could lower dementia risk, others suggest it could increase the risk. However, 'Many of the studies looking at HRT have used it when menopause is in full swing, or it's a bit too late, so it's hard to really judge its effect on thinking and memory,' Katherine Gray, research grants manager at Alzheimer's Society, tells me. 'Based on the latest research, if your GP is going to advise you to go on HRT, it should be as early as possible, in perimenopause, to get the most benefits,' she adds.

Other possible factors in the dementia gap include sleep disturbances and cardiovascular disease brought on by the menopause, and genetic predispositions found more commonly in women. Sociocultural factors like social isolation, and the ability to mask early symptoms through strong verbal skills, may also play a role. The long and the short of it, though, is that much more research is needed to fully understand sex and gender differences in dementia risk and development, as well as the implications for diagnosis and treatment.

It will probably come as no great surprise that dementia research as a whole, as well as research specifically into sex and gender differences, has so far been massively underfunded. It's also worth noting that, despite being disproportionately affected, 2016 research by University College London found that women with dementia receive less medical attention than men.

The Women's Brain Project was founded in 2016 to advance scientific understanding and advocate for women's brain health. Its researchers, along with dementia researchers globally, are now taking steps in the right direction, but there's still a long way to go. Speaking to me in 2019, Dr Laura Phipps from Alzheimer's Research UK said, 'In terms of funding and the discoveries we've been able to make, we're probably a couple of decades behind where cancer is.'

Besides dementia, as we've already mentioned, declining oestrogen at menopause increases the risk of cardiovascular disease – an area where we already know there's a gender gap – and decreases bone density, putting post-menopausal women and AFAB people at increased risk of osteoporosis. An estimated one in two women (compared to one in five men) over 50 will break a bone as a result of osteoporosis, with wrist, hip and spinal fractures particularly common. This becomes increasingly problematic for elderly women, as the risk of falling worsens with age.

Similarly, the loss of oestrogen loosens the supporting structures of the pelvic floor, leading to problems like urinary incontinence and pelvic organ prolapse – or exacerbating existing problems, caused by pregnancy and vaginal birth, which may have gone untreated for decades.

All of these have significant implications for health and social care in later life, which brings us to the other hidden gender disparity: the care gap. According to Carers UK, women make up nearly 60% of the unpaid carers in the UK and are more likely than men to be 'sandwich carers', caring for young children and elderly parents at the same time. Notably, much of this care falls to women at just the time when they're dealing with the onset of their own menopause.

One in four women aged 50–64 has caring responsibilities for older or disabled loved ones, while women aged 45–54 are more than twice as likely as men to have given up work and four times more likely to have reduced their hours to care for others.

It was particularly insulting, then, when in October 2021 then health secretary Sajid Javid suggested that families (read: women) should take responsibility for health and social care, rather than the state. Whether as patients or carers, or both, the reality for far too many menopausal women is an expectation that they'll simply get on with it, taking responsibility for their own health and the health of their loved ones. They, just as much as anyone, deserve better from our healthcare system.

YOUR MENOPAUSE TOOLKIT

If you're struggling with perimenopause or post-menopausal symptoms, one of the best things you can do is track those symptoms, just as you may already track your period. This not only helps you to identify and understand what's going on with your body, but will also help you explain any patterns or ongoing issues to your GP. The Balance app, developed by menopause specialist Dr Louise Newson, has a facility for you to track symptoms or you can simply make notes in a paper diary.

It's also important to understand the risks and benefits of HRT so you can have an informed conversation with your doctor, says Dr Nighat Arif. 'Dr Louise Newson and Diane Danzebrink break this down on their websites, Newson Health and Menopause Support [see page 236], and Dr Avrum Bluming's book *Oestrogen Matters* explains that oestrogen is not carcinogenic. If you have it through the skin, it just tops up what your body is deficient in,' she explains. 'Equally though, there are alternatives out there as well if you can't or don't want to have it.'

Once you feel suitably informed, make an appointment with your GP, taking with you a list or diary of your symptoms. If you haven't had time to track your symptoms, Menopause Support has a symptom checker list on their website, which you can print out and fill in. If you've decided you want to try HRT, Nighat recommends being upfront about this: 'Go to the doctor and say, "I am a menopausal woman. These are my symptoms. I know antidepressants are not a first-line treatment. I would like to try hormone replacement therapy."'

It may be helpful, Diane adds, to print out and take along either a summary of the NICE guidelines or the British Menopause Society's advice for doctors. Bear in mind, too, that if they're not already well informed, they may wish to take this information away and digest it before booking another appointment to talk through treatment options with you.

If you're still not getting anywhere, remember that you're entitled to see someone else. 'Go back to reception and ask if there's a GP in the practice who is, not necessarily a menopause specialist, but at least menopause-aware or with a special interest in women's health,' Diane says. If there's absolutely no one who's clued up, you could ask for a referral to a local menopause clinic, but be aware there may be a long waiting list and your nearest clinic may be many miles away. Alternatively, try presenting the same information to a different GP, who may be more sympathetic and receptive than the first.

Finally, get connected with support services and peer support groups who can offer advice and help you feel less alone with whatever you're going through. If you're also caring for others during this challenging time, remember that it's vital to take good care of yourself as well and it's not selfish to put yourself first every once in a while.

Resources
- Alzheimers Research UK – alzheimersresearchuk.org
- Alzheimers Society – alzheimers.org.uk or call the Dementia Connect support line on 0333 150 3456
- Black Women in Menopause – twitter.com/BLKmeno pause

- British Heart Foundation – bhf.org.uk
- British Menopause Society – thebms.org.uk
- Carers UK – carersuk.org
- Dementia UK – dementiauk.org
- Latte Lounge – lattelounge.co.uk
- Menopause Support – menopausesupport.co.uk
- Menopause Whilst Black – instagram.com/menopau sewhilstblack
- Newson Health – newsonhealth.co.uk
- Queer Menopause – queermenopause.com
- Royal Osteoporosis Society – theros.org.uk
- The Menopause Charity – themenopausecharity.org
- Women's Brain Project – womensbrainproject.com
- Women's Health Concern (patient information from the British Menopause Society) – womens-health -concern.org

11

'Can I speak to a real doctor?': Dismantling a sexist medical model

As I write this, in October 2021, we are more than 18 months into the global Covid-19 pandemic and I am six months pregnant with my first child. Personally, with three months to go until I have to push a baby out of my vagina, I'm staring down the barrel of a midwifery crisis that's been building for months. In the time since I conceived, the number of midwives working in England fell by almost 300 in just two months – the fastest drop in over 20 years. Meanwhile, findings from the RCM revealed a terrifying 57% of midwives are considering leaving within the next year. This is, the *Metro* reports, 'In part due to understaffing and fears that they cannot offer safe care to women in the current system.' In my local hospital, short-staffing in recent months has led to an increase in negative birth experiences being reported. Maybe I just know too much about everything that can go wrong, but I'm scared.

Meanwhile, every single ambulance service in the country is on the highest level of alert, with paramedics reporting that patients are waiting in ambulances outside hospitals for up to 11 hours before being seen in A&E. In the community, GPs are on the receiving end of a sustained attack by both the government and right-wing press over access to face-to-face appointments, despite having seen an enormous increase in their workload since the pandemic began. They're tired. Many are leaving what is already a critically understaffed workforce. In 2015, then health secretary Jeremy Hunt pledged to expand the GP workforce by 5000 by 2020, but the reality in 2021 is that GP numbers have dropped by nearly 1400 instead, not helped by the pressures of the pandemic.

'It might not look like GPs are busy, but it's definitely much busier behind the scenes. Since the pandemic I've gone from having 30 to 35 patient contacts on a bad day to now having 50 on an average day. It's really challenging,' Dr Katie Cairns, a GP based in Northern Ireland, tells me. 'Telephone triage means many more patients can access same-day telephone appointments with us, instead of waiting weeks to see us in person, but it definitely hasn't made my working life any easier.'

Tensions are high. A growing number of patients are frustrated and fed up with the struggle to be seen in person. They're anxious about their own and their families' health. They're tired of feeling that all other healthcare has apparently been 'put on hold', although the truth is that healthcare professionals are doing their utmost to keep things moving along. Meanwhile, staff are understandably exhausted, burnt out and at their wits' end.

It feels like this relationship has reached boiling point. Hospitals have been vandalised and doctors have been attacked. In July 2021 the BMA reported that 37% of doctors had experienced verbal abuse in the past month, and more than half had witnessed violence or abuse against other staff. These figures rose significantly in general practice, where 51% of GPs had been abused in the previous month, one in five reported being threatened, and 67% said their experience of abuse, threatening behaviour and violence had got worse over the last year.

It's certainly a far cry from the early days of the pandemic, when everyone hung rainbows in their windows, clapped and banged pans for our 'NHS heroes' every Thursday night. Conversations about the NHS now feel divisive. Covid-19 cases continue to rise and hospitals are rapidly filling up again as we hurtle towards a winter fourth wave. The NHS and the government's scientific advisors are calling for restrictions to be reintroduced before it's too late, but there seems to be little public or political appetite for it. The healthcare professionals I speak to are frightened, while the government and the public appear to be living in a blissful state of denial. It all feels a bit too much like déjà vu.

None of this is how I'd planned to start this final chapter. But it's a difficult context in which to have a nuanced or compassionate conversation about problems in the healthcare system and it feels important to acknowledge the challenges that exist on both sides of the battle lines that are being drawn.

Earlier in 2021, charity Engage Britain published a UK-wide survey into patient experiences. It found that 77% of the 4000 people surveyed were proud of the NHS and 85% 'acknowledged that NHS staff are overstretched, doing as much as they can with the resources available.' However, one in five had resorted to seeking private care because of NHS failings, one in four said waiting times had harmed their mental health and 28% felt they 'had to fight for treatment.' More than a quarter of patients felt their problems were not taken seriously – and, you won't be surprised to hear, that figure rose to 45% among women aged 18–34. Meanwhile, 22% of people from ethnic minorities said they or a loved one had experienced racism when seeking treatment.

Several high-profile doctors reacted defensively on Twitter, accusing Engage Britain of attacking the NHS and acting as mouthpieces for those in the Conservative Party who are set on its privatisation. If anything, in my view, it did the opposite. It highlighted exactly why we need to fight so hard to save our NHS for the benefit of all patients; to oppose the increasing sell-off and privatisation-by-stealth of NHS services; and to demand adequate funding from a government that has consistently underfunded it for more than a decade.

What it also made clear, though, is that there's a problem around how we critique the system. How can we unpick it, rebuild it, reform it, without ultimately losing something that is so important to all of us? And, of course, how can we separate the Covid fallout from the problems that existed long beforehand?

Almost all the patient stories I've included here, and certainly all the problems I've described, pre-date the pandemic. Many of them stem from global issues, like medical misogyny and bias in scientific research – areas in which the UK healthcare system is far from unique. It is worth noting, though, that the UK has the largest gender health gap in the G20 and the 12th largest in the world. In her *First Do No Harm* report, which I discussed in chapters 1, 6 and 8, Baroness Julia Cumberlege writes that our healthcare system is: 'disjointed, siloed, unresponsive and defensive. It does not adequately recognise that patients are its *raison d'etre*. It has failed to listen to their concerns and when, belatedly, it has decided to act it has too often moved glacially.' The strain that Covid-19 has placed on the system, and the subsequent disruption to routine healthcare services, have only made matters worse.

Yet so much of this was not inevitable. It was the result of many years' worth of political choices that have stripped our NHS to its bones and left it on its knees. Recovery will be a long and challenging process, both for the system as a whole and for all those staff who have been battered and bruised by their pandemic experiences. But demanding better care and reduced inequality is not at odds with fiercely, passionately defending our NHS and supporting its workers.

The gender health gap revolution – and each individual act of patient advocacy that makes it up – which I've detailed in these pages has been described as a medical #MeToo movement; a mass speaking out of women and others about the biases and mistreatment they have faced. It's not a perfect analogy by any stretch, but it's perhaps useful as a way of thinking about the broader structural, patriarchal issues at play, and how we might begin to dismantle them, together, as patients and as healthcare professionals.

Taken piece by piece, my work often reads as a catalogue of individual failings by individual doctors who – whether through ignorance, arrogance, policy or prejudice – let their patients down. But I hope that, taken as a whole, it paints a picture of a flawed system in which the vast majority of healthcare professionals are simply trying their best with what they have available to them. Throughout this book, and my broader work, I've looked to the wisdom, compassion, experience and expertise of many doctors, nurses, midwives and other health workers, and I've seen the constraints and challenges that they, too, face when it comes to navigating the healthcare profession.

*

Seventy-seven per cent of the NHS workforce are women – including 89% of nurses and health visitors, just under 50% of all doctors and more than 50% of GPs. Data from NHS Digital shows that, between 2009 and 2017, the number of female hospital and community health service doctors increased by nearly 11,000, while the number of male doctors rose by just over 4000. Forty-six per cent of medical staff are non-white, around 3% of NHS staff are openly lesbian, gay or bisexual and, although trans status isn't centrally recorded, the NHS Trans Staff Network has more than 170 members from across the profession.

But a diverse workforce is not necessarily an equal workforce. While women and ethnic minorities are well represented in junior and frontline roles, they remain significantly outnumbered by white men in more senior roles, both clinical and non-clinical: 64% of consultants, for example, are men and almost 60% are white. And, just as we've seen patients come up against sexism, racism, ableism, homophobia, transphobia and other biases within healthcare, staff from marginalised groups face similar challenges going about their everyday work.

A report published by the BMA in August 2021 revealed that more than 90% of female doctors had experienced sexism at work in the past two years, with 61% feeling discouraged from working in a particular specialty because of their gender and 70% believing their clinical ability had been doubted or undervalued because of their gender. More than half the women surveyed said they'd experienced unwanted verbal comments relating to their gender, while one in three had experienced 'unwanted physical conduct' in their place of work.

The report states that, despite the significant increase in women joining medicine in recent decades, too many people still view it as a male profession. 'The failure to address structures and policies that favour a workforce of men, allowing sexist attitudes and gender bias to remain prevalent, has led to unequal opportunities for women,' it says. 'Sexism is impacting women's long-term career progression and causing problems in their day-to-day working lives.'

Meanwhile, the 2020 survey of all (clinical and non-clinical) NHS staff found that, in the previous 12 months, 17% of ethnic minority staff, 12% of gay or lesbian staff and 13% of bisexual staff had experienced discrimination from a manager, team leader or other colleagues. So had 13% of those with a long-term health condition and 9% of those with childcare responsibilities. Meanwhile, 19% of ethnic minority staff, 14% of gay or lesbian staff and 12% of bisexual staff had experienced discrimination from patients, relatives or other members of the public. Of the more than 400,000 women who reported experiencing discrimination at work, 23% said this discrimination was on the basis of their gender and 46% said it was because of their ethnic background.

'As Black women in medicine, people see us as less competent, less qualified. If we speak up we are stereotyped as "angry Black women". People assume we don't speak English or they mock our accents,' Dr Omon Imohi tells me in an interview for Hysterical Women. Omon is a Nigerian-born NHS GP and founder of Black Women in Healthcare, a network inspired by her own experience of feeling overlooked when she started her NHS training. 'There is already gender bias and inequality in medicine, before you bring in race, so as a Black woman you are doubly disadvantaged and discriminated against,' she adds.

Most shockingly, Omon tells me about one Black, female junior doctor being dismissed by a nurse who asked to speak to 'a real doctor' instead. 'Comments like that are really hurtful and if there are healthcare professionals who will treat their Black colleagues like that, how will they speak to Black patients?' she says.

Writing for the *BMJ*, Dr Rageshri Dhairyawan, a consultant in sexual health and HIV medicine, describes being mistakenly treated as a more junior member of staff during her redeployment to Covid-19 wards in 2020, while more junior colleagues were treated as the consultant. Though she initially put her discomfort about the situation down to imposter syndrome, she writes: 'I now see that perhaps this wasn't imposter phenomenon that I was experiencing, but rather a credibility deficit. There may well have been instances where I was perceived to not fit the stereotype of what a consultant looks like, whilst my white and male registrars did.'

Chatting to me later, Rageshri reflects on another experience, this time as a patient undergoing IVF treatment, when fellow medics dismissed her pain, framing her as a nuisance and a drug-seeker despite her professional status as a consultant. 'That experience, as a woman of colour having my pain dismissed, was really eye-opening. Even though I was a doctor, who knew what was going on and how to advocate for myself, I was struck by the power imbalance and how vulnerable you are as a patient,' she says.

'We still rely on stereotypes quite a bit in medicine and I think a lot of that goes back to what we're taught in medical school. When we're in situations where we have to make decisions quickly, sometimes those mental shortcuts can be useful, but we do need to be aware that these stereotypes may not always be right and that we might be using them wrongly,' she tells me.

'I'm an Asian woman and one of the stereotypes, particularly about older Asian women, is that they ache all over – not necessarily because they're in pain, but because of anxiety or other emotional reasons. That's a stereotype that links back to the idea of hysteria and it's one we really need to challenge. But we're not taught about the history of women and pain in our training or how racial bias can impact on whether or not doctors prescribe painkillers,' Rageshri explains.

'It shouldn't really take the experience of being a patient for me and other doctors to think about things like this, but I think other, systemic, issues come in here, too. We don't get much time with our patients, and the less time we have the more likely we are to rely on mental shortcuts and stereotypical views of the patient in front of us. The pressures within the system make it hard for doctors to really take the time to reflect,' she adds.

*

For both Omon and Rageshri, these personal and professional experiences directly mirror what so many women of colour report as patients – feelings of being dismissed, disbelieved, not taken as seriously as their white male counterparts. The same is true of the ableism that's embedded within the healthcare profession. GP trainee Dr Hannah Barham-Brown, who uses a wheelchair to manage the pain caused by EDS, has seen first-hand some of the attitudes to disability that exist within the healthcare profession.

'I made a very conscious, thought-through decision to get a wheelchair when I did, but I've had a number of health professionals tell me that was the wrong thing to do,' she says. 'I have a very physical job that I cannot do without ending up exhausted and in pain unless I use the chair. For me it's a pain management method and it enables me to live an independent life, but I think there's a big attitude in medicine that if you don't need a wheelchair, why would you want to use one? That comes from a real misunderstanding around what "needing a wheelchair" is,' she explains.

Similarly, Hannah adds, 'I've worked in GP surgeries where I could not get my wheelchair through the door of my own clinic room. I scraped the paint off the doorframe getting in and out every day. If I can't get in, how am I able to care for patients who are in wheelchairs or mums with buggies? Equally, I've turned up at sexual health clinics as a patient and found they're up two flights of stairs, and it's like, oh, this is because I obviously don't have sex, right?'

For her, the challenges of being a disabled doctor were particularly acute during her time working in hospitals. 'When you're a junior in hospital medicine, the expectations and requirements are vast, and the pressures are different. You've got to be dashing around a hospital, juggling multiple lever arch files, while steering a wheelchair. When you're also being bombarded with more work than one team can possibly take on, who you're working with is really important. I'm not trying to defend my former colleagues, who made my life a bit of a misery, but I can see how the pressure means that, if you see someone in your team as a weak link, that's going to be frustrating for you,' she explains.

'The best colleagues are the ones who go, "Yes, you work differently, but you bring a whole load of interesting knowledge and experience, and our patients like you." The worst have been the ones who go, "Oh god, I'm on with her. I'm going to be doing the running round. I'm going to be carrying things. She's never going to keep up." Nine times out of ten, I've more than kept up – in fact, I can go very, very fast in a wheelchair – but they don't see it like that. They don't see my working differently as being potentially a good thing; they see it as another burden on them.'

It's notable, too, that the number of LGB staff who are out at work varies quite significantly from region to region, with some NHS Trusts recording just 1–2% of their staff as gay, lesbian or bisexual, while others report that LGB staff make up 7–8% of their workforce. 'One of the biggest issues we see is staff not feeling consistently able to be out. Maybe being out to their line manager and some local colleagues, but not other wider colleagues, or being out to colleagues but not their manager,' explains Tara Hewitt, who has worked in equality lead roles for the NHS for over a decade, including as associate director of inclusion & engagement at the Northern Care Alliance, one of the biggest NHS organisations in the country.

Tara is also one of the most senior trans women currently working in the NHS and founder of the NHS Trans Staff Network. 'Many of the trans people I know in the NHS felt like they were the only trans person in their organisation. Particularly if you're in a more junior role, you don't want to be known as the trans nurse or the trans porter and a lot of people felt that if they spoke up about inequalities or shared their story at work they would be viewed in that way,' she says.

'There's almost a feeling of being grateful for having a job and being supported by their line manager, and not wanting to rock the boat. The idea with the staff network was to allow some of those stories to be shared anonymously. When issues have come up I've been able to share those examples of inequalities to help improve services and decision-making, where there wouldn't otherwise have been a trans voice included.'

For frontline trans staff, Tara says experiences are very similar to the kind of discrimination she hears about from LGB and ethnic minority colleagues, many of whom feel powerless to challenge the abuse that's directed at them at work. 'A lot of people from marginalised communities who go into healthcare come from a position of "I'm here to help, it doesn't matter if someone's being horrible to me or shouting abuse, I'm still going to try and help." That makes me so sad,' she says.

'We have seen a number of NHS organisations make it clear that, no matter how unwell someone is, if they're choosing to abuse our colleagues then those colleagues should be empowered and supported to not feel they have to continue delivering care,' Tara adds. 'We've also had a number of Trust chief execs and senior leaders come out publicly and say, "We will not tolerate transphobia or any forms of discrimination." But more consistency of this approach is needed across the country, with actions rather than words leading the way.'

*

Policy change in the NHS is notoriously glacial and risk-averse. There are good reasons for this when it comes to providing cost-effective, evidence-based healthcare, but it's a frustrating way of tackling long-standing inequalities, particularly when those responsible for policy change aren't representative of the patients they serve.

'The NHS as an institution is often focused on incremental rather than transformational change. You might have a policy review, where you tweak things and change a line, but you rarely scrap the policy and completely rewrite it,' Tara explains. The under-representation of marginalised groups in those decision-making roles is where bias often comes in, she adds: 'When you look at the history of the NHS, there's a legacy of gender inequality in leadership, and we're still seeing the drip-through of that history.' Likewise, the absence of LGBTQ+ people, disabled people and people of colour from these roles means issues affecting these groups are not necessarily considered – and this, as we've seen in so many different ways, is reflected in the service as a whole.

While this kind of top-down representation has improved somewhat over the last 70 years, there's still a long way to go for truly representative senior leadership in the NHS. In the meantime, though, the patient advocacy I've documented here will remain vital for shifting the agenda. Healthcare professionals, too, have an important role to play and many of them are just as engaged in their own forms of activism – from sharing engaging and accurate health information on Instagram and TikTok, to lobbying for policy changes, and working to encourage diversity and inclusive care in their own workplaces.

Besides working as a trainee GP, Hannah is deputy leader of the Women's Equality Party and regularly speaks out about disability and women's issues within the medical profession. 'I've done a big piece of work around cervical screening and the complete lack of hoists for disabled women who are hoist-dependent. That's a really big problem, but I don't think I'd know about it if I wasn't a disabled doctor, and the British Medical Association wouldn't know about it had I not got up at a conference and said: "You do realise that hoist-dependent women are struggling to get cervical screening, right?" People just don't think about it,' she explains.

'That's not anything malicious or negligent, it's just not on their radar at all. So often we don't even know where the gaps in our knowledge are. That's one of the reasons I work so bloody hard to try and get more disabled medical students and doctors into the profession, because that's how we improve things,' Hannah adds.

During my conversations with doctors, another common theme has been the need for medical school curricula to properly address health inequalities and medical bias. 'We need to place greater importance in medical school on communication skills and how our implicit biases may impact on individuals' care,' says consultant obstetrician Dr Christine Ekechi.

'I think all medical professionals need to have some level of education about the history of Western modern medicine, because it's vitally important to understand where medicine has gone wrong, not redo things we've done before, and progress in an ethical way,' adds sexual health doctor Annabel Sowemimo, who founded Decolonising Contraception.

For her, addressing racial biases in medical education includes practical examples like understanding how dermatology symptoms present on darker skin tones, as well as a more fundamental reckoning with medicine's racist and colonial past. This history, she explains, has inevitably had an impact on relations with racially minoritised patient groups and must be addressed in order to understand how the healthcare profession can better serve these patients going forwards.

One of the positives I've heard from several doctors, though, is an optimism that broader cultural shifts are beginning to filter through. There's a general feeling that, even if curricula haven't changed much yet, the next generation of medical students are more feminist, actively anti-racist, inclusive and understanding of LGBTQ+ patients than previous generations. It's a good reason to feel hopeful – providing, that is, that all the acceptance and compassion isn't crushed out of them by the ever-increasing pressures of the job.

'The system is broken and it's not sustainable,' Omon tells me. 'We've been underfunded and understaffed for years. In general practice that means there aren't enough appointments for patients and GPs have increasing workloads. Each appointment is limited to 10 minutes, so patients feel rushed, but if you run over it throws off your whole day. Some GPs are still at the practice at 7 or 8 o'clock in the evening trying to catch up from everything and it's these issues that are causing burnout.'

While GP, ambulance and A&E services have been the most visibly affected, chronic understaffing and staff burnout is an increasing problem across the board. A 2021 BMA survey found that nearly 80% of doctors have experienced 'moral distress' – defined as: 'the psychological unease generated where professionals identify an ethically correct action to take but are constrained in their ability to take that action' – while working through the pandemic. This rose to almost 90% among doctors from ethnic minority backgrounds.

The biggest factors contributing to moral distress were having insufficient staff to suitably treat all patients, followed by mental fatigue, lack of time to emotionally support patients and inability to provide timely treatments. When asked what could help alleviate their moral distress, almost 60% of respondents said, quite simply: 'More staff.' Figures from NHS Digital show that there were more than 93,000 full-time equivalent vacancies across the NHS in June 2021, the highest number recorded since December 2019. Staffing issues were particularly acute in nursing, an overwhelmingly female profession – which is to say, one that's notoriously underpaid and undervalued.

This staffing crisis doesn't just harm all healthcare professionals' ability to do their jobs with the required levels of empathy, care and attention; it's an existential threat to the entire future of the NHS. In that rather bleak context, where on earth do we go from here when it comes to tackling the gender health gap?

*

At the most fundamental level, we need a properly functioning health service. That requires funding for necessary equipment and infrastructure, but above all it requires people – well-trained, compassionate, skilled people and plenty of them. Adequate staffing levels are essential for patient safety and we urgently need investment, not just in recruiting more doctors, nurses, midwives and support staff, but also ensuring they're well enough paid and supported to do their jobs to the best of their abilities, and to keep them in those roles long-term.

We need these staff to be diverse, inclusive and trained in recognising and challenging their own biases and those of their colleagues. This type of awareness and self-reflection must become ingrained in medical school curricula and other healthcare training courses, but it should also be an ongoing part of continuing professional development and lifelong learning. We need to rethink the medical model that still too often views textbook knowledge as fixed, infallible and in conflict with patients' own intimate knowledge of themselves; to drop the idea that 'doctor knows best' and instead begin to treat medicine as a collaborative partnership between patients and healthcare professionals, each with complementary forms of expertise. The patient-centred 'ICE' model for medical consultations is a great starting point, and already widely used. Introduced by Pendelton *et al* in 1984, it's based on exploring patients' ideas, concerns and expectations, with the aim of achieving a shared understanding.

We need those in management to be truly representative of all the staff and patients the NHS serves, and to consider the healthcare needs of all patient groups when making decisions about policy and service planning. That includes working with marginalised patients to develop strategies that take real, tangible steps towards tackling health inequalities, rather than simply paying lip service to 'equality and diversity' or dismissing these groups as 'hard to reach'.

We need research to bridge the many gaps in medical knowledge, and to inform more effective treatments and diagnostic tools. As we've seen there are dozens of female-dominant health issues, across all sorts of medical specialities, all desperately vying for a sliver of research funding and attention. It's difficult to know where to even begin with filling in these gaps, but, if you're a budding researcher, a quick flick back through these pages should offer plenty of potential starting points.

Growing numbers of women in medicine and research will no doubt help, but the major problem, as always, is money. We need a concerted funding effort to support research in fields like menstrual and reproductive health, menopause, autoimmunity and chronic pain. We also need medical researchers across all fields to properly consider the implications of sex and gender in their work, as well as overlapping factors like race, socioeconomic background and trans status, even when it comes to seemingly gender-neutral issues.

Finally, we need the results of that newfound medical knowledge to trickle down, not only to those healthcare professionals currently in training, but to anyone whose patients could benefit. Medical science must continue to change, grow and evolve in this way, and we need healthcare professionals to adapt their existing practice when presented with new evidence, rather than stubbornly persisting with the way they've always done things.

Throughout this book we've already seen how powerful and important patient advocacy can be. Even during these most challenging of times for the NHS, sustained pressure from campaigners has thrust issues like menopause and the Black maternal mortality rate onto the political and public agenda. Similarly, Long Covid activism has shone a light on the experiences of those with other long-neglected chronic illnesses, and conversations about conditions like endometriosis have continued to gain media attention. There is a real momentum here and, regardless of how bleak healthcare in the UK feels right now, I also can't help but feel a little bit hopeful for the future.

Part of that hopefulness comes from my passionate and long-held belief in the power of sisterhood, solidarity and women coming together to make change happen. These women have been the central voices in my work, not only because their stories deserve to be heard, but because they really can and do help to make a difference. I also feel hopeful about the number of healthcare professionals still fighting for change in the face of such enormous pressure and uncertainty. The very best of these are informed not just by their own compassion and professional expertise, but by listening to their patients.

Of course, none of the changes I've outlined here can happen overnight or without significant investment and reform. The gender health gap is a stubborn, patriarchal beast and there is an awful lot of hard work to be done at institutional levels to tackle it. In truth, it's this systemic stuff I'm least hopeful about – the changes that will require our government to invest vast sums of money and commit to radical policy transformations rather than decades more of tinkering around the edges. I'm certainly not naive enough to believe that, even collectively, individual patients and clinicians can fix a centuries-old problem like medical misogyny. But what we can do is continue to shift attitudes in the right direction and chip away at the most egregious examples.

That said, some political momentum is already underway, as we've seen. In the decade since I started writing about these issues, patient advocacy has already led to policy changes like the scrapping of the tampon tax, and the addition of both menstrual and menopause education to school curriculums, as well as relationships, sex and health education being made mandatory for the first time. All Party Parliamentary Groups have been established to investigate issues in areas including endometriosis, ME and menopause care, and the government has commissioned reviews and inquiries into a number of high-profile women's health scandals, although tangible action from these has so far been less forthcoming.

For all the harm done by the pandemic, it did strengthen the case for a rethink about the way healthcare – particularly when it comes to sexual and reproductive health – operates. We can see this with the increased momentum towards self-sampling pilots for cervical screening, the move to pharmacists carrying out contraceptive pill checks, and the reclassification of two types of contraceptive (progesterone-only) 'mini pills' allowing them to be sold over the counter. Most significant, though, was the emergency Covid measure that successfully introduced telemedical abortion services in England, Wales and Scotland. A review of this scheme found that allowing women to access reproductive health consultations from home, and to be sent abortion pills by post if clinically appropriate, was 'safe, effective, and preferable for many women'. Following a public consultation, MPs voted in March 2022 to make this permanent, representing an important step forward for reproductive health.

There's no room for complacency though, as recent events across the Atlantic demonstrate. The Supreme Court's decision to overturn Roe v Wade – removing the federal right to an abortion in the US – sent shockwaves across the globe. It's worth remembering that, while the political context is very different, abortion is still governed by criminal law in England, Scotland and Wales. This makes it unlike any other medical procedure, with patients and healthcare professionals facing prosecution if abortions are not carried out in line with the 1967 Abortion Act. Meanwhile in Northern Ireland, where abortion was decriminalised in 2019, there is still no way of accessing an abortion because of an ongoing lack of service provision. Clearly, we can't take anything for granted, and the campaign for decriminalisation across the rest of the UK feels more vital than ever.

Meanwhile, in 2021 Scotland became the first country in the UK to set out a Women's Health Plan, with key actions including the appointment of a national Women's Health Champion and a Women's Health Lead in every NHS board, and the establishment of a Women's Health Research Fund to close gaps in scientific and medical knowledge. Over the border in England, there was also a landmark government consultation on women's healthcare experiences. The findings, from more than 100,000 responses, were stark – but won't come as much of a surprise after everything you've already read: 84% of respondents reported feeling that they had not been listened to by healthcare staff and nearly two-thirds of those with a long-term health condition or disability felt they weren't adequately supported.

This consultation helped to inform the Department of Health and Social Care's new Women's Health Strategy for England, published in July 2022. This too included pledges on improving research and the appointment of a Women's Health Ambassador, Professor Dame Lesley Regan – a former president of the Royal College of Obstetricians and Gynaecologists (RCOG), who brings to the role a wealth of experience and expertise. The landmark strategy also promises the introduction of mandatory teaching and assessment on women's health for medical students and new doctors; the removal of barriers to IVF for same-sex couples; and improved access to high-quality health information and education. Significantly, from my perspective, it acknowledges that women's health goes beyond the 'bikini medicine' of breast health and gynaecology, with references to autism, dementia, mental health, cardiovascular health and long-term physical illness and disability – although nothing specifically on female-dominant conditions like ME or fibromyalgia.

However, there's also much that still feels quite vague and non-committal, and concerns have been raised about the apparent lack of new investment to fund the ambitions laid out in the strategy. On endometriosis diagnosis times, for example, there is a 10-year ambition that: 'women and girls with severe endometriosis experience better care, where diagnosis time is reduced' – yet it's unclear what is meant by 'severe', or what the plan is for patients with 'non-severe' disease, and there is no specific target for how much diagnosis time should be reduced by. Similarly, the strategy promises to 'encourage' the expansion of one-stop Women's Health Hubs – yet it's apparent that this will need to be funded from within existing budgets. Reacting to the strategy's publication, then president of the RCOG Dr Edward Morris said: 'We are… concerned at the lack of dedicated funding to make these ambitions a reality. Confirmed funding to support the instrumental changes the strategy sets out is lacking and, with existing budgets already being stretched further each year, it will mean that progress will be slow for vital initiatives like women's health hubs.' Grassroots campaigners have also expressed concerns about the government's commitment to inclusion, diversity and co-production for under-served communities, including women of colour, trans and non-binary patients.

These issues will have to be addressed going forwards, but it is welcome news that many of the right conversations are at least being had – even if progress feels frustratingly slow. Much of the political rhetoric is broadly promising, but it will be meaningless unless it's backed up by the government putting its money where its mouth is on funding for research and services.

Either way, these conversations show no sign of slowing down, shutting up or going away. My hope is that they will become more and more collaborative – dialogues between patients and healthcare professionals based on mutual empathy and trust, not dismissiveness or resentment. This will, by necessity, involve hearing and acknowledging some uncomfortable truths. Doctors will have to accept that the way they've always done things may have been wrong or harmful. They'll have to get better at admitting they don't have all the answers and facing up to what that means for their practice. Many will have to reflect on biases that influence the way they treat their patients, and reassess the stereotypes they rely on to make clinical judgements and decisions each day.

As patients, too, we need to recognise – but not accept – the limitations of the current, broken system and continue demanding the powers that be do something about it. We need to learn how best to work within the system, alongside the professionals who care for us, and when and how advocating for ourselves might be useful. Above all, we need to continue speaking out whenever and wherever possible – complaining, expecting better, pushing for research and policy change, and the kind of care we all ultimately deserve.

Our rebellious, unruly bodies have been ignored and neglected for long enough. Misunderstood and stigmatised because they're too female, too dark, too broken, too fat, too old, too young, too trans or too queer. Dismissed as hormonal and irrational. Written off as hysterical, as mad, as liars. But rest assured that the fightback is on and every rebel body has a part to play.

REFERENCES

1. 'THE PERSONAL IS POLITICAL': INTRODUCTION

Germaine Greer famously encouraged women to taste their own menstrual blood: Greer, G., 1970. *The Female Eunuch*. London: MacGibbon & Kee.

the landmark women's health publication *Our Bodies, Ourselves*: The Boston Women's Health Book Collective, 1976. *Our Bodies, Ourselves*. Boston, Mass.: Simon & Schuster.

The title of a 1970 Carol Hanisch essay, 'the personal is political' highlights the intersection between personal experience and broader socio-political contexts: ThoughtCo. 2020. *The Personal Is Political: Where Did the Feminist Slogan Come From?* [online] Available at: <https://www.thoughtco.com/the-personal-is-political-slogan-origin-3528952> [Last accessed 8 August 2022].

in the words of Black feminist scholar Kimberlé Williams Crenshaw, 'The process of recognising as social and systemic what was formerly perceived as isolated and individual': Crenshaw, K., 1991. Mapping the Margins: Intersectionality, Identity Politics, and Violence against Women of Color. *Stanford Law Review*, 43(6), p.1241.

endometriosis alone is estimated to cost the UK economy £8.2 billion a year: Endometriosis-uk.org. *Endometriosis Facts and Figures | Endometriosis UK*. [online] Available at: <https://www.endometriosis-uk.org/endometriosis-facts-and-figures> [Last accessed 8 August 2022].

14 million working days per year are lost to the menopause: Papadatou, A. and Papadatou, A., *Menopause costs UK economy 14 million working days per year – HRreview*. [online] HRreview. Available at: <https://www.hrreview.co.uk/hr-news/menopause-costs-uk-economy-14-million-working-days-per-year/115754> [Last accessed 8 August 2022].

women are up to three times more likely than men to die from a heart attack: Alabas, O., Gale, C., Hall, M., Rutherford, M., Szummer, K., Lawesson, S., Alfredsson, J., Lindahl, B. and Jernberg, T., 2017. Sex Differences in Treatments, Relative Survival, and Excess Mortality Following Acute Myocardial Infarction: National Cohort Study Using the SWEDEHEART Registry. *Journal of the American Heart Association*, 6(12).

Black women are four times more likely than white women to die in childbirth: Knight, M., Bunch, K., Tuffnell, D., Patel, R., Shakespeare, J., Kotnis, R., Kenyon, S., Kurinczuk, J.J. (Eds.) on behalf of MBRRACE-UK. Saving Lives, Improving Mothers' Care – Lessons learned to inform maternity care from the UK and Ireland Confidential Enquiries into Maternal Deaths and Morbidity 2017-19. Oxford: National Perinatal Epidemiology Unit, University of Oxford 2021.

On the origins of 'hysteria': Micale, M.S., 2019. *Approaching Hysteria: Disease and Its Interpretations*. Princeton: Princeton University Press.

'Since their sole purpose was to bear and raise children, women's health was entirely defined by their uteruses': Cleghorn, E., 2021. *Unwell Women: A journey through myth and medicine in a man-made world*. London: Weidenfeld & Nicolson.

Freud's Studies on Hysteria helped to establish the still-persistent association between hysteria and so-called 'conversion' or 'psychosomatic' disorders: Freud, S. and Breuer, J., 1974. *Studies on hysteria*. Harmondsworth: Penguin.

removed from the standard US clinical handbook, Diagnostic and Statistical Manual of Mental Disorders: Tasca, C., Rapetti, M., Carta, M. G., & Fadda, B. (2012). Women and hysteria in the history of mental health. *Clinical practice and epidemiology in mental health: CP & EMH, 8*, pp.110–119.

Black patients 22% less likely than white patients to be prescribed pain medication: Meghani, S., Byun, E. and Gallagher, R., 2012. Time to Take Stock: A Meta-Analysis and Systematic Review of Analgesic Treatment Disparities for Pain in the United States. *Pain Medicine*, 13(2), pp.150-174.

A US study as recently as 2016 found that half of white medical students held false beliefs: Hoffman, K., Trawalter, S., Axt, J. and Oliver, M., 2016. Racial bias in pain assessment and treatment recommendations, and false beliefs about biological differences between blacks and whites. *Proceedings of the National Academy of Sciences*, 113(16), pp.4296-4301.

Similar experiences are documented by Baroness Julia Cumberlege: Cumberlege, J., 2020. *First Do No Harm – The report of the Independent Medicines and Medical Devices Safety Review*. [online] Available at: <https://www.immdsreview.org.uk/downloads/IMMDSReview_Web.pdf> [Last accessed 8 August 2022].

Writing for the Guardian in 2013 about #TransDocFail, journalist Jane Fae asked: Fae, J., 2013. *The real trans scandal is not the failings of one doctor but cruelty by many.* [online] The Guardian. Available at: <https://www.theguardian.com/commentisfree/2013/jan/10/trans-scandal-doctor-richard-curtis-transdocfail> [Last accessed 8 August 2022].

by our conversation, I founded Hysterical Women, a trans-inclusive feminist health blog: *Hysterical Women.* [online] Available at: <https://hystericalwomen.co.uk/> [Last accessed 8 August 2022].

A 2017 report by the King's Fund… states that: "The NHS is under growing financial pressure...': Robertson, R., Wenzel, L., Thompson, J. and Charles, A., 2017. *Understanding NHS financial pressures: how are they affecting patient care?* [online] The King's Fund. Available at: <https://www.kingsfund.org.uk/publications/understanding-nhs-financial-pressures> [Last accessed 8 August 2022].

According to a report by the doctors' professional body, the British Medical Association (BMA), published in July 2020, much of this was 'avoidable': BMA, 2020. *The hidden impact of COVID-19 on patient care in the NHS in England.* [online] BMA. Available at: <https://www.bma.org.uk/media/2841/the-hidden-impact-of-covid_web-pdf.pdf> [Last accessed 8 August 2022].

2. 'SOME GIRLS JUST HAVE BAD PERIODS': MENSTRUAL AND HORMONAL HEALTH

One in every 5000 girls will be born with Mayer Rokitansky Küster Hauser syndrome (MRKH): MRKH Connect. *What is MRKH?* [online] Available at: <https://mrkhconnect.co.uk/what-is-mrkh/> [Last accessed 8 August 2022].

one in 10,000 girls and young women will be affected by premature ovarian insufficiency (POI): The Daisy Network. *What is POI.* [online] Available at: <https://www.daisynetwork.org/about-poi/what-is-poi/> [Last accessed 8 August 2022].

feminist Gloria Steinem imagines a world in which only men have periods: Steinem, G., 2019. If Men Could Menstruate (Article Reprint). *Women's Reproductive Health*, 6(3), pp.151-152.

more than 50% of young women experience period pain bad enough to need medication: Grandi, G., Ferrari, Xholli, Cannoletta, Palma, Volpe and Cagnacci, A., 2012. Prevalence of menstrual pain in young women: what is dysmenorrhea? *Journal of Pain Research*, p.169.

medications used to treat period pain… have a 20-25% failure rate: Proctor, M., Latthe, P., Farquhar, C., Khan, K. and Johnson, N., 2005. Surgical interruption of pelvic nerve pathways for primary and secondary dysmenorrhoea. *Cochrane Database of Systematic Reviews*, 2010(11).

researchers conduct five times as many studies into erectile dysfunction (ED) as PMS, despite the former affecting just 19% of men while the latter, in varying forms, affects 90% of women: ResearchGate. 2016. *Why do we still not know what causes PMS?* [online] Available at: <https://www.researchgate.net/blog/why-do-we-still-not-know-what-causes-pms> [Last accessed 8 August 2022].

An earlier review found that 40% of women with PMS do not respond to any of the currently available treatments: Freeman, E., 2010. Therapeutic management of premenstrual syndrome. *Expert Opinion on Pharmacotherapy*, 11(17), pp.2879-2889.

Endometriosis is the second most common gynaecological condition: Endometriosis-uk.org. *Endometriosis Facts and Figures | Endometriosis UK.* [online] Available at: <https://www.endometriosis-uk.org/endometriosis-facts-and-figures> [Last accessed 8 August 2022].

endometriosis and other female-dominant conditions are among the worst funded by the US National Institutes of Health: Mirin, A., 2021. Gender Disparity in the Funding of Diseases by the U.S. National Institutes of Health. *Journal of Women's Health*, 30(7), pp.956-963.

As recently as 2017 the National Institute of Health and Care Excellence (NICE) published its first guidance on endometriosis: Boseley, S., 2017. *'Listen to women': UK doctors issued with first guidance on endometriosis.* [online] The Guardian. Available at: <https://www.theguardian.com/society/2017/sep/06/listen-to-women-uk-doctors-issued-with-first-guidance-on-endometriosis> [Last accessed 8 August 2022].

'Historically, endometriosis was perceived as a "white women's disease"': Chatman, D., 1976. Endometriosis in the black woman. *American Journal of Obstetrics and Gynecology*, 125(7), pp.987-989.

PCOS, a condition that affects around one in ten women and AFAB people... more than 50% of people with PCOS won't have any symptoms: NHS. *Polycystic ovary syndrome.* [online] Available at: <https://www.nhs.uk/conditions/polycystic-ovary-syndrome-pcos/> [Last accessed 8 August 2022].

women with PCOS are more likely to be diagnosed with depression, anxiety or bipolar: Berni, T., Morgan, C., Berni, E. and Rees, D., 2018. Polycystic Ovary Syndrome Is Associated With Adverse Mental Health and Neurodevelopmental Outcomes. *The Journal of Clinical Endocrinology & Metabolism*, 103(6), pp.2116-2125.

pre-menstrual dysphoric disorder (PMDD), is estimated to affect 5-8% of women and people who menstruate: NAPS – National Association for Premenstrual Syndromes. *About PMS.* [online] Available at: <https://www.pms.org.uk/about-pms/> [Last accessed 8 August 2022].

books like Emma Barnett's: Barnett, E., 2019. *Period: It's About Bloody Time.* London: HQ.

and Maisie Hill's: Hill, M., 2019. *Period Power.* London: Green Tree.

During the launch of a report from the All-Party Parliamentary Group (APPG) on Endometriosis in October 2020...: Graham, S., 2020. *Blaming women for being 'fobbed off' shows the Government doesn't take endometriosis seriously.* [online] The Telegraph. Available at: <https://www.telegraph.co.uk/women/life/blaming-women-fobbed-shows-government-doesnt-take-endometriosis/> [Last accessed 8 August 2022].

waiting lists for gynaecology increased by 60% during the pandemic: The Guardian. 2022. *Dismissal of women's health problems as 'benign' leading to soaring NHS lists.* [online] Available at: <https://www.theguardian.com/society/2022/jun/02/dismissal-of-womens-health-problems-as-benign-leading-to-soaring-nhs-lists> [Last accessed 8 August 2022].

3. 'ATTENTION-SEEKING HYPOCHONDRIACS': THE GENDER PAIN GAP

'The girl who cried pain: A bias against women in the treatment of pain': Hoffmann, D. and Tarzian, A., 2001. The Girl Who Cried Pain: A Bias Against Women in the

Treatment of Pain. [online] Available at: <https://ssrn.com/abstract=383803> [Last accessed 8 August 2022].

women in pain are kept waiting longer in A&E than men: Robertson, J., 2014. *Waiting Time at the Emergency Department from a Gender Equality Perspective*. Gothenberg: Institute of Medicine at the Sahlgrenska Academy, University of Gothenburg.

...less likely to be taken seriously: Hoffmann, D. and Tarzian, A., 2001. The Girl Who Cried Pain: A Bias Against Women in the Treatment of Pain. [online] Available at: <https://ssrn.com/abstract=383803> [Last accessed 8 August 2022].

...less likely to be prescribed opioid painkillers: Chen, E., Shofer, F., Dean, A., Hollander, J., Baxt, W., Robey, J., Sease, K. and Mills, A., 2008. Gender Disparity in Analgesic Treatment of Emergency Department Patients with Acute Abdominal Pain. *Academic Emergency Medicine*, 15(5), pp.414-418.

...more likely to be prescribed sedatives or anti-anxiety medication: Calderone, K., 1990. The influence of gender on the frequency of pain and sedative medication administered to postoperative patients. *Sex Roles*, 23(11-12), pp.713-725.

Black patients half as likely to receive pain medication as white patients: Singhal, A., Tien, Y. and Hsia, R., 2016. Racial-Ethnic Disparities in Opioid Prescriptions at Emergency Department Visits for Conditions Commonly Associated with Prescription Drug Abuse. *PLOS ONE*, 11(8), p.e0159224.

50% of white medical students held at least one false belief about biological differences between races: Hoffman, K., Trawalter, S., Axt, J. and Oliver, M., 2016. Racial bias in pain assessment and treatment recommendations, and false beliefs about biological differences between blacks and whites. *Proceedings of the National Academy of Sciences*, 113(16), pp.4296-4301.

lesbian women, trans and non-binary patients – as well as disabled LGBT people and Black, Asian and minority ethnic LGBT people – were the most likely to experience unequal treatment...: Bachmann, C. and Gooch, B., 2018. *LGBT in Britain – Health*. [online] Stonewall. Available at: <https://www.stonewall.org.uk/system/files/lgbt_in _britain_health.pdf> [Last accessed 8 August 2022].

'marked changes in sex hormones [i.e. through gender-affirming hormone therapy] affect the occurrence of pain' in some, but not all, trans patients: Aloisi, A., Bachiocco, V., Costantino, A., Stefani, R., Ceccarelli, I., Bertaccini, A. and Meriggiola, M., 2007. Cross-sex hormone administration changes pain in transsexual women and men. *Pain*, 132(Supplement 1), pp.S60-S67.

'...the evidence... was surprisingly weak and inconsistent': Hunt, K., Adamson, J., Hewitt, C. and Nazareth, I., 2011. Do women consult more than men? A review of gender and consultation for back pain and headache. *Journal of Health Services Research & Policy*, 16(2), pp.108-117.

gender disparities at every stage of heart attack care: 2019. *Bias and Biology: How the gender gap in heart disease is costing women's lives*. [online] British Heart Foundation. Available at: <https://www.bhf.org.uk/-/media/files/heart-matters/bias-and-biology -briefing.pdf?rev=cd26147a45f9444098aa2949551f3803&hash=7C4225981A8554B 921502F609C42C7F9> [Last accessed 8 August 2022].

women are seven times more likely than men to be misdiagnosed and discharged in the middle of a heart attack: Pope, J., Aufderheide, T., Ruthazer, R., Woolard, R., Feldman, J., Beshansky, J., Griffith, J. and Selker, H., 2000. Missed Diagnoses of Acute Cardiac Ischemia in the Emergency Department. *New England Journal of Medicine*, 342(16), pp.1163-1170.

Although there are some sex differences in symptom presentation, research suggests these are 'modest': DeVon, H., Mirzaei, S. and Zègre-Hemsey, J., 2020. Typical and Atypical Symptoms of Acute Coronary Syndrome: Time to Retire the Terms? *Journal of the American Heart Association*, 9(7).

according to one paper published in 2019, women are more likely than men to experience 'typical' symptoms: Ferry, A., Anand, A., Strachan, F., Mooney, L., Stewart, S., Marshall, L., Chapman, A., Lee, K., Jones, S., Orme, K., Shah, A. and Mills, N., 2019. Presenting

REFERENCES

Symptoms in Men and Women Diagnosed With Myocardial Infarction Using Sex-Specific Criteria. *Journal of the American Heart Association*, 8(17).

'Medical education might have you believe that as future doctors we will solely be treating men...': Politis, M., 2021. *"Mr X presents with central crushing chest pain"—Breaking the male norm in medical education.* [online] The BMJ. Available at: <https://blogs.bmj .com/bmj/2021/07/22/mr-x-presents-with-central-crushing-chest-pain-breaking-the -male-norm-in-medical-education/> [Last accessed 8 August 2022].

coronary heart disease, which causes most heart attacks, is the leading cause of death for women globally: European Society of Cardiology. *Cardiovascular Disease in Women.* [online] Available at: <https://www.escardio.org/The-ESC/Advocacy/women-and -cardiovascular-disease> [Last accessed 8 August 2022].

'non-traditional risk factors' for both heart attack and stroke... are rising more steeply in women than men: Hänsel, M., Steigmiller, K., Luft, A., Gebhard, C., Held, U. and Wegener, S., 2022. Neurovascular disease in Switzerland: 10-year trends show non-traditional risk factors on the rise and higher exposure in women. *European Journal of Neurology*, 29(9), pp.2851-2860.

research shows women are typically slower to go to hospital than men: Bugiardini, R., Ricci, B., Cenko, E., Vasiljevic, Z., Kedev, S., Davidovic, G., Zdravkovic, M., Miličić, D., Dilic, M., Manfrini, O., Koller, A. and Badimon, L., 2017. Delayed Care and Mortality Among Women and Men With Myocardial Infarction. *Journal of the American Heart Association*, 6(8).

A study on 4732 medical students showed that two-thirds of them had conscious, explicit, anti-fat bias and three-quarters had implicit bias: Phelan, S., Dovidio, J., Puhl, R., Burgess, D., Nelson, D., Yeazel, M., Hardeman, R., Perry, S. and Ryn, M., 2014. Implicit and explicit weight bias in a national sample of 4,732 medical students: The medical student CHANGES study. *Obesity*, 22(4), pp.1201-1208.

Studies show that doctors are less inclined to examine fat patients: Phelan, S., Burgess, D., Yeazel, M., Hellerstedt, W., Griffin, J. and Ryn, M., 2015. Impact of weight bias and stigma on quality of care and outcomes for patients with obesity. *Obesity Reviews*, 16(4), pp.319-326.

84% of patients in larger bodies reported that their weight is blamed for most medical problems: Puhl, R. and Heuer, C., 2009. The Stigma of Obesity: A Review and Update. *Obesity*, 17(5), pp.941-964.

A systematic review found that BMI only has a one in three success rate: Tomiyama, A., Hunger, J., Nguyen-Cuu, J. and Wells, C., 2016. Misclassification of cardiometabolic health when using body mass index categories in NHANES 2005–2012. *International Journal of Obesity*, 40(5), pp.883-886.

patients who are overweight – as well as those who smoke – are treated as 'soft targets' for NHS savings: 2016. *Smokers and Overweight Patients: Soft targets for NHS savings?* [online] The Royal College of Surgeons of England. Available at: <https://www.rcseng .ac.uk/library-and-publications/rcs-publications/docs/smokers-soft-targets/> [Last accessed 8 August 2022].

68% of women with high BMIs reported that they delayed seeking healthcare: Puhl, R. and Heuer, C., 2010. Obesity Stigma: Important Considerations for Public Health. *American Journal of Public Health*, 100(6), pp.1019-1028.

...ditching the health service's counterproductive obsession with BMI and instead adopting a 'Health At Every Size' (HAES) approach: Women and Equalities Committee, 2021. *Changing the perfect picture: an inquiry into body image.* [online] House of Commons. Available at: <https://committees.parliament.uk/publications /5357/documents/53751/default/> [Accessed 8 August 2022].

telling trans women they aren't wearing enough lipstick or 'feminine' clothing: The Independent. 2021. *Trans women being told they 'aren't wearing enough lipstick' by doctors, MPs hear.* [online] Available at: <https://www.independent.co.uk/life-style /health-and-families/trans-women-lipstick-healthcare-equality-b1846803.html> [Accessed 8 August 2022].

a third of trans people have experienced some form of unequal treatment: Bachmann, C. and Gooch, B., 2018. *LGBT in Britain – Health*. [online] Stonewall. Available at: <https://www.stonewall.org.uk/system/files/lgbt_in_britain_health.pdf> [Last accessed 8 August 2022].

70% of respondents said they'd experienced some form of transphobia: TransActual. 2021. *Trans lives survey 2021*. [online] Available at: <https://www.transactual.org.uk/trans-lives-21> [Accessed 8 August 2022].

nearly 50% of trans and gender non-conforming patients avoid going to the emergency department: Samuels, E., Tape, C., Garber, N., Bowman, S. and Choo, E., 2018. "Sometimes You Feel Like the Freak Show": A Qualitative Assessment of Emergency Care Experiences Among Transgender and Gender-Nonconforming Patients. *Annals of Emergency Medicine*, 71(2), pp.170-182.e1.

Dr Ben Vincent, a non-binary academic and author of *Transgender Health: A Practitioner's Guide to Binary and Non-Binary Trans Patient Care*: Vincent, B., 2018. *Transgender Health: A Practitioner's Guide to Binary and Non-Binary Trans Patient Care*. Jessica Kingsley.

'Women scored higher than men on measures of patient likelihood to self-advocate': Kolmes, S. and Boerstler, K., 2020. Is There a Gender Self-Advocacy Gap? An Empiric Investigation Into the Gender Pain Gap. *Journal of Bioethical Inquiry*, 17(3), pp.383-393.

4. 'CHRONICALLY FEMALE': WHY DISABILITY IS A FEMINIST ISSUE

women spend more of their lives with poor health and disability: Gender Equality Index 2019. Work-life balance. *Women live longer but in poorer health*. [online] Available at: <https://eige.europa.eu/publications/gender-equality-index-2019-report/women-live-longer-poorer-health> [Last accessed 9 August 2022].

data published by the UK government for the year 2018/19 shows that disability is more prevalent in women (7.7 million) than men (6.3 million): GOV.UK. 2020. *Family Resources Survey: financial year 2018/19*. [online] Available at: <https://www.gov.uk/government/statistics/family-resources-survey-financial-year-201819> [Last accessed 9 August 2022].

Chronic pain is one of the leading causes of disability worldwide, affecting more than a third of the UK population: Fayaz, A., Croft, P., Langford, R., Donaldson, L. and Jones, G., 2016. Prevalence of chronic pain in the UK: a systematic review and meta-analysis of population studies. *BMJ Open*, 6(6), p.e010364.

'Chronic pain affects a higher proportion of women than men…': International Association for the Study of Pain (IASP). *Pain in Women*. [online] Available at: <https://www.iasp-pain.org/advocacy/global-year/pain-in-women/> [Accessed 9 August 2022].

The *Unseen, Unequal, Unfair* report into chronic pain in England: Ellis, B., Ly, M. and Steinberger, S., 2021. *Unseen, Unequal, Unfair: Chronic Pain in England*. [online] Versus Arthritis. Available at: <https://www.versusarthritis.org/media/23739/chronic-pain-report-june2021.pdf> [Accessed 9 August 2022].

Women make up almost 80% of those affected by autoimmune diseases: Fairweather, D. and Rose, N., 2004. Women and Autoimmune Diseases. *Emerging Infectious Diseases*, 10(11), pp.2005-2011.

women also appear to be most affected by the emerging condition… known as Long Covid: The PHOSP-COVID Collaborative Group, 2022. Clinical characteristics with inflammation profiling of long COVID and association with 1-year recovery following hospitalisation in the UK: a prospective observational study. *The Lancet Respiratory Medicine*, 10(8), pp.761-775.

62% of people with autoimmune diseases are labelled 'chronic complainers': Stairs, L., 2021. *Diagnosing Rare Autoimmune Diseases*. [online] Future of Personal Health.

Available at: <https://www.futureofpersonalhealth.com/rare-diseases/the-difficult-road-to-rare-autoimmune-disease-diagnosis/> [Last accessed 16 August 2022].

one study noted higher burdens of disability in trans people than cis people: Downing, J. and Przedworski, J., 2018. Health of Transgender Adults in the U.S., 2014–2016. *American Journal of Preventive Medicine*, 55(3), pp.336-344.

a review of the evidence around chronic disease in transgender populations highlighted 'critical gaps: Rich, A., Scheim, A., Koehoorn, M. and Poteat, T., 2020. Non-HIV chronic disease burden among transgender populations globally: A systematic review and narrative synthesis. *Preventive Medicine Reports*, 20, p.101259.

One literature review concluded that: 'Compared to men, women have more pain: Samulowitz, A., Gremyr, I., Eriksson, E. and Hensing, G., 2018. "Brave Men" and "Emotional Women": A Theory-Guided Literature Review on Gender Bias in Health Care and Gendered Norms towards Patients with Chronic Pain. *Pain Research and Management*, 2018, pp.1-14.

what *Doing Harm* author Maya Dusenbery terms: Dusenbery, M., 2018. *Doing Harm: The Truth About How Bad Medicine and Lazy Science Leave Women Dismissed, Misdiagnosed, and Sick*. New York, NY: HarperOne.

In 2019 Chronically Awesome surveyed nearly 700 members on their experiences: 2020. *Market Research 2019*. [online] Chronically Awesome. Available at: <https://chronicallyawesome.org.uk/wp-content/uploads/2020/03/Chronically-Awesome-Market-Research-2019.pdf> [Last accessed 9 August 2022].

A separate survey of almost 800 disabled women and non-binary people, carried out by Chronic Illness Inclusion (CII) in 2021: 2021. *Submission to the Department of Health and Social Care's Inquiry into Women's Health and Wellbeing in England*. [online] Chronic Illness Inclusion. Available at: <https://chronicillnessinclusion.org.uk/wp-content/uploads/2021/06/CII.DHSC-Womens-Health-England-June-2021.pdf> [Last accessed 9 August 2022].

ME, the long-term, fluctuating, multisystem condition affecting 250,000 people in the UK, an estimated 75-80% of whom are women: #MEAction Network. *What is ME?* [online] Available at: <https://www.meaction.net/learn/what-is-me/> [Last accessed 9 August 2022].

After a review of evidence proved they're ineffective at best: 2020. *Evidence reviews for the nonpharmacological management of ME/CFS*. [online] National Institute for Health and Care Excellence. Available at: <https://www.nice.org.uk/guidance/ng206/documents/evidence-review-7> [Last accessed 9 August 2022].

then health secretary Sajid Javid promised 'radical action' for patients: O'Neill, S., 2022. *Sajid Javid promises radical action for patients debilitated by ME*. [online] The Times. Available at: <https://www.thetimes.co.uk/article/sajid-javid-promises-radical-action-for-patients-debilitated-by-me-9bkq6qf5g> [Last accessed 9 August 2022].

NICE published updated guidelines on the treatment of unexplained chronic pain: 2021. *Chronic pain (primary and secondary) in over 16s: assessment of all chronic pain and management of chronic primary pain*. NICE guideline. [online] National Institute for Health and Care Excellence. Available at: <https://www.nice.org.uk/guidance/ng193/resources/chronic-pain-primary-and-secondary-in-over-16s-assessment-of-all-chronic-pain-and-management-of-chronic-primary-pain-pdf-66142080468421> [Last accessed 9 August 2022].

genetic correlations between endometriosis and a number of inflammatory autoimmune conditions: Shigesi, N., Kvaskoff, M., Kirtley, S., Feng, Q., Fang, H., Knight, J. C., Missmer, S. A., Rahmioglu, N., Zondervan, K. T., & Becker, C. M. (2019). The association between endometriosis and autoimmune diseases: a systematic review and meta-analysis. *Human reproduction update*, 25(4), 486–503.

fibromyalgia, which causes chronic widespread pain, may in fact be an autoimmune response: Goebel, A., Krock, E., Gentry, C., Israel, M., Jurczak, A., Urbina, C., Sandor, K., Vastani, N., Maurer, M., Cuhadar, U., Sensi, S., Nomura, Y., Menezes, J., Baharpoor, A., Brieskorn, L., Sandström, A., Tour, J., Kadetoff, D., Haglund, L., Kosek, E., Bevan,

S., Svensson, C. and Andersson, D., 2021. Passive transfer of fibromyalgia symptoms from patients to mice. *Journal of Clinical Investigation*, 131(13).

DecodeME project is set to be the largest ever biomedical study of ME: DecodeME. *Get Involved*. [online] Available at: <https://www.decodeme.org.uk/> [Last accessed 9 August 2022].

'Viral infections prompt the immune system to respond...': The Guardian. 2021. *Why are women more prone to long Covid?* [online] Available at: <https://www.theguardian.com /society/2021/jun/13/why-are-women-more-prone-to-long-covid> [Last accessed 9 August 2022].

it's suggested that 'Sex hormones may further amplify this hyperimmune response...': Fairweather, D. and Rose, N., 2004. Women and Autoimmune Diseases. *Emerging Infectious Diseases*, 10(11), pp.2005-2011.

our fluctuating hormone cycles were deemed too complicated: Liu, K. and DiPietro Mager, N., 2016. Women's involvement in clinical trials: historical perspective and future implications. *Pharmacy Practice*, 14(1), pp.708-708.

Black and ethnic minority backgrounds were at disproportionate risk of serious illness or death from Covid-19: 2020. *Disparities in the risk and outcomes of COVID-19*. [online] Public Health England. Available at: <https://assets.publishing.service.gov.uk/ government/uploads/system/uploads/attachment_data/file/908434/Disparities_in_the _risk_and_outcomes_of_COVID_August_2020_update.pdf> [Last accessed 9 August 2022].

disabled women with higher support needs were 91% more likely to die from Covid-19. Disabled people more generally had a 'markedly increased' risk of mortality from Covid: Bosworth, M., Ayoubkhani, D., Nafilyan, V., Foubert, J., Glickman, M., Davey, C. and Kuper, H., 2021. Deaths involving COVID-19 by self-reported disability status during the first two waves of the COVID-19 pandemic in England: a retrospective, population-based cohort study. *The Lancet Public Health*, 6(11), pp.e817-e825.

the Care Quality Commission (CQC) found that 30% of people with a DNR order in place were not aware of it: 2021. *Protect, respect, connect – decisions about living and dying well during COVID-19*. [online] Care Quality Commission. Available at: <https://www .cqc.org.uk/sites/default/files/20210318_dnacpr_printer-version.pdf> [Last accessed 9 August 2022].

Scope reported 63% of disabled people were concerned they wouldn't get the hospital treatment: Scope. 2020. *Disabled people and the coronavirus crisis*. [online] Available at: <https://www.scope.org.uk/campaigns/disabled-people-and-coronavirus/the-disability -report/> [Last accessed 9 August 2022].

In 2007 it published Death by Indifference: 2007. *Death by indifference*. [online] Mencap. Available at: <https://www.mencap.org.uk/sites/default/files/2016-06/DBIreport.pdf> [Last accessed 9 August 2022].

followed up a decade later by its current, ongoing Treat Me Well campaign: Mencap. *Treat Me Well*. [online] Available at: <https://www.mencap.org.uk/get-involved/campaign -mencap/treat-me-well> [Last accessed 9 August 2022].

The 2018 Learning Disabilities Mortality Review found the median age at death for people with learning disabilities: 2018. *Annual Report*. The Learning Disability Mortality Review (LeDeR) Programme. [online] University of Bristol Norah Fry Centre for Disability Studies. Available at: <https://www.hqip.org.uk/wp-content/uploads/2019/05 /LeDeR-Annual-Report-Final-21-May-2019.pdf> [Last accessed 9 August 2022].

Pre-Covid, in 2018, Mencap estimated that 1200 learning disabled people each year died avoidably: Mencap, 2018. *Concerns over lack of clinical training causing avoidable learning disability deaths*. [online] Available at: <https://www.mencap.org.uk/press -release/concerns-over-lack-clinical-training-causing-avoidable-learning-disability -deaths> [Last accessed 9 August 2022].

According to charity PoTS UK, up to 50% of patients are told their symptoms are 'all in their head': Kavi, L., Nuttall, M., Low, D., Opie, M., Nicholson, L., Caldow, E. and Newton, J., 2016. A profile of patients with postural tachycardia syndrome and their experience of healthcare in the UK. *British Journal of Cardiology*, 23.

As of March 2021, Kelly and Asad were two of more than 100,000 NHS employees affected by Long Covid: The Guardian. 2021. *Strain on NHS as tens of thousands of staff suffer long Covid*. [online] Available at: <https://www.theguardian.com/society /2021/apr/03/nhs-feels-strain-tens-thousands-staff-long-covid> [Last accessed 9 August 2022].

5. 'ALL IN YOUR HEAD': MENTAL HEALTH AND HYSTERIA

In the 2005 edition of her 1972 book *Women and Madness*, Phyllis Chesler writes: 'In my time...': Chesler, P., 2018. *Women and Madness*. Chicago: Lawrence Hill Books, p.1.

Drs Paula J Caplan and Lisa Cosgrove point out in their 2004 book *Bias in Psychiatric Diagnosis*: Cosgrove, L. and Caplan, P., 2004. *Bias in Psychiatric Diagnosis*. Lanham MD: Jason Aronson.

Women are more likely than men to be diagnosed with common mental health issues like depression and anxiety: McManus S, Bebbington P, Jenkins R, Brugha T. Mental health and wellbeing in England: Adult Psychiatric Morbidity Survey 2014 [online]. Available at: <https://webarchive.nationalarchives.gov.uk/ukgwa/20171010183932tf_/http:// content.digital.nhs.uk/catalogue/PUB21748/apms-2014-full-rpt.pdf> [Last accessed 9 August 2022].

...as well as eating disorders: Beat. *Statistics for Journalists*. [online] Available at: <https:// www.beateatingdisorders.org.uk/media-centre/eating-disorder-statistics/> [Last accessed 9 August 2022].

...and PTSD: Tolin, D. and Foa, E., 2006. Sex differences in trauma and posttraumatic stress disorder: A quantitative review of 25 years of research. *Psychological Bulletin*, 132(6), pp.959-992.

The controversial diagnosis of borderline or emotionally unstable personality disorder (BPD/EUPD) is overwhelmingly applied to women: Skodol, A. and Bender, D., 2003. Why Are Women Diagnosed Borderline More Than Men? *Psychiatric Quarterly*, 74(4), pp.349-360.

Black patients are disproportionately diagnosed with stigmatised conditions like schizophrenia: Schwartz, R., 2014. Racial disparities in psychotic disorder diagnosis: A review of empirical literature. *World Journal of Psychiatry*, 4(4), p.133.

Psychiatric medication like antidepressants and anti-anxiety drugs are also more likely to be prescribed to women: Boyd, A., Van de Velde, S., Pivette, M., ten Have, M., Florescu, S., O'Neill, S., Caldas-de-Almeida, J., Vilagut, G., Haro, J., Alonso, J. and Kovess-Masféty, V., 2015. Gender Differences in Psychotropic Use Across Europe: Results From a Large Cross-Sectional, Population-Based Study. *European Psychiatry*, 30(6), pp.778-788.

men are believed to be more likely than women to under-report their struggles with mental ill health... self-medicating using recreational drugs and alcohol, or expressing their emotions in more physical ways like violence and aggression: Smith, D., Mouzon, D. and Elliott, M., 2016. Reviewing the Assumptions About Men's Mental Health: An Exploration of the Gender Binary. *American Journal of Men's Health*, 12(1), pp.78-89.

mental ill health among women is on the rise: McManus S, Bebbington P, Jenkins R, Brugha T. Mental health and wellbeing in England: Adult Psychiatric Morbidity Survey 2014 [online]. Available at: <https://webarchive.nationalarchives.gov.uk/ukgwa /20171010183932tf_/http://content.digital.nhs.uk/catalogue/PUB21748/apms-2014 -full-rpt.pdf> [Last accessed 9 August 2022].

29% of Black women, 24% of Asian women and 29% of mixed-race women affected by common mental health problems: 2017. *Race Disparity Audit*. [online] Cabinet Office. Available at: <https://assets.publishing.service.gov.uk/government/uploads/system/ uploads/attachment_data/file/686071/Revised_RDA_report_March_2018.pdf> [Last accessed 9 August 2022].

staggeringly high rates of depression and anxiety, particularly among lesbian and bisexual women, trans and non-binary people: Bachmann, C. and Gooch, B., 2018. *LGBT in*

Britain – Health. [online] Stonewall. Available at: <https://www.stonewall.org.uk/system/files/lgbt_in_britain_health.pdf> [Last accessed 8 August 2022].

Women who experience sexism are more likely to develop mental health issues: Hackett, R., Steptoe, A. and Jackson, S., 2019. Sex discrimination and mental health in women: A prospective analysis. *Health Psychology*, 38(11), pp.1014-1024.

As Daniel and Jason Freeman, authors of *The Stressed Sex*, note: 'Social stresses make people vulnerable to mental illness: Freeman D., Freeman J., 2013. *The stressed sex: Uncovering the truth about men, women, and mental health.* Oxford: Oxford University Press.

Women are also twice as likely as men to have experienced trauma from interpersonal violence and abuse: Scott, S. and McManus, S., 2016. *Hidden Hurt: Violence, abuse and disadvantage in the lives of women.* [online] Agenda. Available at: <https://weareagenda.org/wp-content/uploads/2015/11/Hidden-Hurt-full-report1.pdf> [Last accessed 9 August 2022].

Campaigns like CALM (the Campaign Against Living Miserably) have been influential in highlighting these issues: The Campaign Against Living Miserably (CALM), 2016. *Record male suicide awareness as new stats show 3 in 4 UK suicides are men.* [online] Available at: <https://www.mynewsdesk.com/uk/calm/pressreleases/record-male-suicide-awareness-as-new-stats-show-3-in-4-uk-suicides-are-men-1678227> [Last accessed 9 August 2022].

although men are more likely to die from their attempts, women actually attempt suicide at higher rates: Schrijvers, D., Bollen, J. and Sabbe, B., 2012. The gender paradox in suicidal behavior and its impact on the suicidal process. *Journal of Affective Disorders*, 138(1-2), pp.19-26.

in 2019, the suicide rate for women and girls was at its highest since 2004: Iacobucci, G. Suicide rates continue to rise in England and Wales. *BMJ* 2020;370:m3431.

patients with severe mental illnesses – including eating disorders, bipolar disorder and PTSD – were left waiting up to two years: Royal College of Psychiatrists, 2020. *Two-fifths of patients waiting for mental health treatment forced to resort to emergency or crisis services.* [online] Available at: <https://www.rcpsych.ac.uk/news-and-features/latest-news/detail/2020/10/06/two-fifths-of-patients-waiting-for-mental-health-treatment-forced-to-resort-to-emergency-or-crisis-services> [Last accessed 9 August 2022].

Black British adults experience the most severe mental health symptoms, they're the least likely to receive treatment – yet are four times more likely to be detained (sectioned): 2018. *Racism and mental health: position statement.* [online] Royal College of Psychiatrists. Available at: <https://www.rcpsych.ac.uk/pdf/PS01_18a.pdf> [Last accessed 9 August 2022].

regard trans people's mental health as relevant only in terms of or in relation to transition,' writes Dr Ruth Pearce, author of *Understanding Trans Health*: Pearce, R., 2018. *Understanding Trans Health: Discourse, power and possibility.* Bristol: Policy Press.

As one 2019 *Guardian* article explains: 'BPD and complex PTSD are different disorders: The Guardian. 2019. *Are sexual abuse victims being diagnosed with a mental disorder they don't have?* [online] Available at: <https://www.theguardian.com/lifeandstyle/2019/mar/27/are-sexual-abuse-victims-being-diagnosed-with-a-mental-disorder-they-dont-have> [Accessed 9 August 2022].

looked at overlapping behaviour treats of people diagnosed with BPD and autism: Dudas, R., Lovejoy, C., Cassidy, S., Allison, C., Smith, P. and Baron-Cohen, S., 2017. The overlap between autistic spectrum conditions and borderline personality disorder. *PLOS ONE*, 12(9), p.e0184447.

both autism and ADHD are significantly under-diagnosed in women and girls: Rudra, A., 2022. *Why many women with autism and ADHD aren't diagnosed until adulthood – and what to do if you think you're one of them.* [online] The Conversation. Available at: <https://theconversation.com/why-many-women-with-autism-and-adhd-arent

-diagnosed-until-adulthood-and-what-to-do-if-you-think-youre-one-of-them
-179970> [Last accessed 9 August 2022].

the gender ratio of autistic males to females, for example, suggest rates ranging from 2:1
to 16:1, with 3:1 currently considered the most up-to-date estimate: National Autistic
Society. *Autistic women and girls.* [online] Available at: <https://www.autism.org.uk
/advice-and-guidance/what-is-autism/autistic-women-and-girls> [Last accessed 9
August 2022].

42% of women and girls had been diagnosed with psychiatric, personality or eating
disorders prior to receiving their autism diagnosis, compared to 30% of men and boys:
2012. *The way we are: autism in 2012.* The National Autistic Society.

Similarly with ADHD, girls are more likely to demonstrate 'inattentiveness': Quinn, P. and
Madhoo, M., 2014. A Review of Attention-Deficit/Hyperactivity Disorder in Women
and Girls: Uncovering This Hidden Diagnosis. *The Primary Care Companion For CNS
Disorders.*

an estimated 1.25 million people in the UK have an eating disorder: Beat. *Statistics for
Journalists.* [online] Available at: <https://www.beateatingdisorders.org.uk/media
-centre/eating-disorder-statistics/> [Last accessed 9 August 2022].

the prevailing stereotype prevents BAME, LGBT+ and people from less affluent
backgrounds from seeking and receiving medical treatment: Beat Eating Disorders,
2019. *New research shows eating disorder stereotypes prevent people finding help.*
[online] Available at: <https://www.beateatingdisorders.org.uk/news/beat-news/eating
-disorder-stereotypes-prevent-help/> [Accessed 9 August 2022].

6. 'CAN YOU GET A PENIS IN AND A BABY OUT?' THE PLEASURE GAP IN SEXUAL AND REPRODUCTIVE HEALTH

You can see this in what's been dubbed the 'gender orgasm gap': Frederick, D., John, H.,
Garcia, J. and Lloyd, E., 2017. Differences in Orgasm Frequency Among Gay, Lesbian,
Bisexual, and Heterosexual Men and Women in a U.S. National Sample. *Archives of
Sexual Behavior*, 47(1), pp.273-288.

44% of women couldn't identify the vagina… while 60% didn't know what the vulva
(external genitalia) was: HuffPost UK. 2016. *Nearly Half Of Women Can't Identify
The Vagina, So How Can They Spot Cancer?* [online] Available at: <https://www
.huffingtonpost.co.uk/entry/half-of-women-cannot-identify-vagina-eve-appeal-survey
_uk_57c6e0f7e4b085cf1ecccea5.> [Last accessed 9 August 2022].

a 2013 review of medical textbooks found a distinct lack of accurate information about
normal, healthy female genitalia: Andrikopoulou, M., Michala, L., Creighton, S.
and Liao, L., 2013. The normal vulva in medical textbooks. *Journal of Obstetrics and
Gynaecology*, 33(7), pp.648-650.

the detailed anatomy of the clitoris was first depicted in the 19th century, it wasn't until
2005 that this information became more widely known: O'Connell, H., Sanjeevan, K.
and Huton, J., 2005. Anatomy of the Clitoris. *Journal of Urology*, 174(4 Pt 1), pp.1189-
1195.

cis women are nearly five times as likely as cis men to feel not listened to: Eve Appeal,
2021. *Nearly five times more women than men have felt 'not listened to' when seeking
medical help for their reproductive health.*

female sexual dysfunction (FSD) is estimated at 41% worldwide: McCool-Myers, M.,
Theurich, M., Zuelke, A., Knuettel, H. and Apfelbacher, C., 2018. Predictors of female
sexual dysfunction: a systematic review and qualitative analysis through gender
inequality paradigms. *BMC Women's Health*, 18(1).

Fran Bushe, author of *My Broken Vagina*, tells me she heard very similar things from the
doctors she interviewed: Bushe, F., 2021. *My Broken Vagina: One woman's quest to fix
her sex life, and yours.* London: Hodder & Stoughton.

Research shows women typically see at least three doctors before they get a diagnosis
of vulvodynia and 40% never get a diagnosis: Harlow, B. L., & Stewart, E. G.

(2003). A population-based assessment of chronic unexplained vulvar pain: have
we underestimated the prevalence of vulvodynia? *Journal of the American Medical
Women's Association (1972)*, 58(2), 82–88.

More than 80% of people affected by UTIs are women: Bono, M., Leslie, S. and Reygaert,
W., 2022. Urinary Tract Infection. *StatPearls Publishing LLC*.

with 50-60% of all women likely to develop at least one in their lifetime: Al-Badr, A. and
Al-Shaikh, G., 2013. Recurrent Urinary Tract Infections Management in Women: A
Review. *Sultan Qaboos University Medical Journal*, 13(3), pp.359-367.

author of *Cystitis Unmasked*, James tells me: Malone-Lee, J., 2021. *Cystitis Unmasked*. tfm
Publishing Limited.

the urine culture test is 'not fit for purpose': The Guardian. 2018. *UTI test often fails to
detect infection, say researchers*. [online] Available at: <https://www.theguardian.com
/society/2018/dec/12/researchers-call-for-new-uti-urinary-tract-infections-testing
-method> [Last accessed 15 August 2022].

A review of 624 patient outcomes by the Lower Urinary Tract Symptoms clinic in Hornsey:
Swamy, S., Barcella, W., De Iorio, M., Gill, K., Khasriya, R., Kupelian, A., Rohn, J. and
Malone-Lee, J., 2018. Recalcitrant chronic bladder pain and recurrent cystitis but
negative urinalysis: What should we do? *International Urogynecology Journal*, 29(7),
pp.1035-1043.

As recently as March 2022, in response to pressure from campaigners, the NHS updated
its online patient information to include chronic UTIs for the first time: Dimsdale,
C., 2022. *NHS finally recognises chronic urinary tract infections exist in online advice
for patients*. [online] inews.co.uk. Available at: <https://inews.co.uk/news/chronic-uti
-infections-nhs-finally-recognises-debilitating-condition-exists-campaign-1512368>
[Last accessed 15 August 2022].

there's clear evidence within the medical community that the hormones in the pill can, in
some women, cause depression and anxiety: Skovlund, C., Mørch, L., Kessing, L. and
Lidegaard, Ø., 2016. Association of Hormonal Contraception With Depression. *JAMA
Psychiatry*, 73(11), p.1154.

Condoms are 98% effective with perfect use, but only 82% effective with typical use: nhs.u
k. *How effective is contraception at preventing pregnancy?* [online] Available at: <https://
www.nhs.uk/conditions/contraception/how-effective-contraception/> [Last accessed
15 August 2022].

fertility awareness methods… have an estimated 76-88% efficacy with typical use:
Planned Parenthood. *Fertility Awareness Methods*. [online] Available at: <https://www
.plannedparenthood.org/learn/birth-control/fertility-awareness> [Last accessed 15
August 2022].

certain groups experience pressure to accept long-acting reversible contraceptive (LARC)
methods: British Pregnancy Advisory Service; Decolonising Contraception; Division
of Health Research, Lancaster University; Shine Aloud UK, 2021. *Long-acting reversible
contraception in the UK*. [online] British Pregnancy Advisory Service. Available at:
<https://www.bpas.org/media/3477/larc-report-final-laid-up.pdf> [Last accessed 15
August 2022].

the mid-90s 'pill panic', which saw a 25% increase in births and a 9% increase in abortion
rates: Foran, T., 2015. *Don't panic about the pill – it's safer than driving to work*. [online]
The Conversation. Available at: <https://theconversation.com/dont-panic-about-the
-pill-its-safer-than-driving-to-work-42325> [Last accessed 15 August 2022].

7. 'THE WAR ON CANCER': GENDERING THE C WORD

One in two of us will get cancer in our lifetime: Cancer Research UK. *Cancer risk statistics*.
[online] Available at: <https://www.cancerresearchuk.org/health-professional/cancer
-statistics/risk> [Last accessed 15 August 2022].

breast cancer – the most common cancer in women – consistently receives more research
funding in the UK than any other cancer: National Cancer Research Institute. *Spend*

by Research & Disease Site. [online] Available at: <https://www.ncri.org.uk/how-we
-work/cancer-research-database/spend-by-research-category-and-disease-site/> [Last
accessed 15 August 2022].

the research funding is not applied proportionately: The Independent. 2014. *Why do
some forms of cancer receive more research funding than others?* [online] Available at:
<https://www.independent.co.uk/life-style/health-and-families/health-news/why-do
-some-forms-of-cancer-receive-more-research-funding-than-others-9771396.html>
[Last accessed 15 August 2022].

47% of the cancers that people are diagnosed with and 55% of the cancers that people die
from are rare cancers: Cancer52. [online] Available at: <https://www.cancer52.org.uk/>
[Last accessed 15 August 2022].

prevents three-quarters of cases of cervical cancer, saving an estimated 5000 lives each
year: Jo's Cervical Cancer Trust. *Barriers to cervical screening among 25-29 year olds*.
[online] Available at: <https://www.jostrust.org.uk/about-us/our-research-and-policy
-work/our-research/barriers-cervical-screening-among-25-29-year-olds> [Last
accessed 15 August 2022].

reality TV star Jade Goody's death from cervical cancer, aged just 27, was credited with
prompting an extra 400,000 women to go for screening: Lancucki, L., Sasieni, P.,
Patnick, J., Day, T. and Vessey, M., 2012. The impact of Jade Goody's diagnosis and
death on the NHS Cervical Screening Programme. *Journal of Medical Screening*, 19(2),
pp.89-93.

feminists 'saw the speculum as an instrument of power that physicians used against
women,' according to researcher Margarete Sandelowski: Sandelowski, M., 2000. 'This
Most Dangerous Instrument Propriety, Power, and the Vaginal Speculum. *Journal of
Obstetric, Gynecologic & Neonatal Nursing*, 29(1), pp.73-82.

two-thirds of the physically disabled women they surveyed had been unable to access
cervical screening: Jo's Cervical Cancer Trust, 2019. *"We're made to feel invisible"
Barriers to accessing cervical screening for women with physical disabilities*. [online] Jo's
Cervical Cancer Trust. Available at: <https://www.jostrust.org.uk/sites/default/files/jos
_physical_disability_report_0.pdf> [Last accessed 15 August 2022].

just 19% of women with a learning disability or autism had had a recent smear test:
Dimensions and Books Beyond Words, 2018. *#MyGPandMe: Making primary care fair*.
[online] Dimensions. Available at: <https://dimensions-uk.org/wp-content/uploads
/MyGPandMe-Making-primary-car-fair-Dimensions.pdf> [Last accessed 15 August
2022].

around 1% of women in the UK are affected by lichen sclerosus…: British Association of
Dermatologists. *One in five women with a vulval health condition contemplate self-harm
or suicide*. [online] Available at: <https://www.bad.org.uk/one-in-five-women-with-a
-vulval-health-condition-contemplate-self-harm-or-suicide/> [Last accessed 15 August
2022].

only around 5% of those cases will develop into vulval cancer: 2018. *LICHEN SCLEROSUS
in Females*. [online] British Association of Dermatologists. Available at: <https://cdn
.bad.org.uk/uploads/2021/12/29200259/Lichen-Sclerosus-Female-Update-February
-2018-Lay-reviewed-November-20172-1.pdf> [Last accessed 15 August 2022].

Trans women, for example, are 48 times more at risk of breast cancer than cis men, but
three times less at risk than cis women: inews.co.uk. 2021. *'My brother died of ovarian
cancer - we need to increase importance of trans health screening'*. [online] Available
at: <https://inews.co.uk/news/long-reads/ian-duncan-deputy-speaker-house-lords
-interview-brother-died-ovarian-cancer-1125221> [Accessed 15 August 2022].

33% of respondents had experienced pain during or after sex…: Jo's Cervical Cancer Trust,
2019. *Not so simple: The impact of cervical cell changes and treatment*. [online] Jo's
Cervical Cancer Trust. Available at: <https://www.jostrust.org.uk/sites/default/files/jos
_trust_a4_report_spreads_05-6-19-compressed.pdf> [Last accessed 15 August 2022].

men with prostate cancer given advanced robotic surgery: Adams, T., 2018. *The robot
will see you now: could computers take over medicine entirely?* [online] The Guardian.
Available at: <https://www.theguardian.com/technology/2018/jul/29/the-robot-will

-see-you-now-could-computers-take-over-medicine-entirely> [Last accessed 15 August 2022].

review published by the *BMJ* in 2018 concluded that most CIN2 changes, particularly in younger women, get better by themselves: Tainio, K., Athanasiou, A., Tikkinen, K., Aaltonen, R., Cárdenas, J., Hernándes, Glazer-Livson, S., Jakobsson, M., Joronen, K., Kiviharju, M., Louvanto, K., Oksjoki, S., Tähtinen, R., Virtanen, S., Nieminen, P., Kyrgiou, M. and Kalliala, I., 2018. Clinical course of untreated cervical intraepithelial neoplasia grade 2 under active surveillance: systematic review and meta-analysis. *BMJ*, p.k499.

in 2014, just 154 of those women had cryopreservation: Abdallah, Y., Briggs, J., Jones, J., Horne, G. and Fitzgerald, C., 2017. A nationwide UK survey of female fertility preservation prior to cancer treatment. *Human Fertility*, 21(1), pp.27-34.

Dr Cheryl Fitzgerald, a consultant in reproductive medicine at St Mary's, said: 'There is a huge inequity: Allen, V., 2017. *Women cancer patients being denied the chance of a family*. [online] Mail Online. Available at: <https://www.dailymail.co.uk/health/article-4100344/4-female-cancer-patients-eggs-embryos-frozen-treatment.html> [Last accessed 15 August 2022].

8. 'BABY BLUES': PERINATAL CARE AND THE PRICE OF MOTHERHOOD

Rebecca Schiller… reflects on her time as a doula in her book *Why Human Rights in Childbirth Matter*: Schiller, R., 2016. *Why Human Rights in Childbirth Matter*. London: Pinter & Martin.

all of which contribute to the estimated 30,000 traumatic births each year in the UK: Birth Trauma Association. [online] Available at: <https://www.birthtraumaassociation.org.uk/> [Last accessed 15 August 2022].

concerns about NHS maternity units, with 38% of them, at the time of writing, rated as 'requires improvement': Lintern, S., 2020. *Care watchdog to target NHS maternity units after baby death scandals*. [online] The Independent. Available at: <https://www.independent.co.uk/news/health/cqc-maternity-safety-inquiry-baby-deaths-shrewsbury-east-kent-b747195.html> [Last accessed 15 August 2022].

maternity staff at Shrewsbury and Telford Hospital Trust had not listened to mothers: Ockenden, D., 2022. *Findings, conclusions and essential actions from the independent review of maternity services at The Shrewsbury and Telford Hospital NHS Trust*. [online] Gov.uk. Available at: <https://assets.publishing.service.gov.uk/government/uploads/system/uploads/attachment_data/file/1064302/Final-Ockenden-Report-web-accessible.pdf> [Last accessed 15 August 2022].

Black mothers four times more likely than their white counterparts to die during pregnancy and labour: Knight M, Bunch K, Tuffnell D, Patel R, Shakespeare J, Kotnis R, Kenyon S, Kurinczuk JJ (Eds.) on behalf of MBRRACE-UK. Saving Lives, Improving Mothers' Care - Lessons learned to inform maternity care from the UK and Ireland Confidential Enquiries into Maternal Deaths and Morbidity 2017-19. Oxford: National Perinatal Epidemiology Unit, University of Oxford 2021.

70-80% of women experience some nausea and vomiting during pregnancy, HG affects an estimated 1% of those: Pregnancy Sickness Support. *What is Hyperemesis Gravidarum?* [online] Available at: <https://www.pregnancysicknesssupport.org.uk/what-is-hyperemesis-gravidarum/> [Last accessed 15 August 2022].

5% of women with HG end up terminating their pregnancies and more than 50% of them consider it: Nana, M., Tydeman, F., Bevan, G., Boulding, H., Kavanagh, K., Dean, C. and Williamson, C., 2021. Termination of wanted pregnancy and suicidal ideation in hyperemesis gravidarum: A mixed methods study. *Obstetric Medicine*.

women affected by HG are eight times more likely to suffer with anxiety or depression during pregnancy and four times more likely to suffer with postnatal depression: Mitchell-Jones, N., Lawson, K., Bobdiwala, S., Farren, J., Tobias, A., Bourne, T. and

Bottomley, C., 2020. Association between hyperemesis gravidarum and psychological symptoms, psychosocial outcomes and infant bonding: a two-point prospective case–control multicentre survey study in an inner city setting. *BMJ Open*, 10(10).

although women with a higher BMI are twice as likely to have a stillbirth, that risk is still very low: Åmark, H., Westgren, M. and Persson, M., 2018. Prediction of stillbirth in women with overweight or obesity—A register-based cohort study. *PLOS ONE*, 13(11).

An estimated one in four pregnancies end in miscarriage: Tommy's. *How common is miscarriage?* [online] Available at: <https://www.tommys.org/pregnancy-information /im-pregnant/early-pregnancy/how-common-miscarriage> [Last accessed 15 August 2022].

doubling both bereaved parents' risk of depression and quadrupling their risk of suicide: Tommy's, 2021. *Devastating impact of miscarriage laid bare in new research.* [online] Available at: <https://www.tommys.org/about-us/news-views/devastating-impact -miscarriage-laid-bare-new-research> [Last accessed 15 August 2022].

just 0.0086% of women will die in childbirth: Schiller, R., 2016. *Why Human Rights in Childbirth Matter*. London: Pinter & Martin.

an estimated one in three women experience some form of traumatic birth: Reed, R., Sharman, R. and Inglis, C., 2017. Women's descriptions of childbirth trauma relating to care provider actions and interactions. *BMC Pregnancy and Childbirth*, 17(1).

fear of birth is at an all-time high: O'Connell, M., Leahy-Warren, P., Khashan, A., Kenny, L. and O'Neill, S., 2017. Worldwide prevalence of tocophobia in pregnant women: systematic review and meta-analysis. *Acta Obstetricia et Gynecologica Scandinavica*, 96(8), pp.907-920.

Researcher and childbirth activist Beverley Beech, author of *Am I Allowed?*: Beech, B., 2014. Am I Allowed?, AIMS.

'Usually [taking] the form of paternalistic coercion: Beech, B., 2016. Violence in obstetrics. AIMS Journal, 28(2). Available at: https://www.aims.org.uk/journal/item/violence-in-obstetrics [Last accessed September 21, 2022].

the process of requesting a caesarean 'lengthy, difficult or inconsistent...': Birthrights. 2018. *Maternal request caesarean.* [online] Available at: <https://www.birthrights.org .uk/campaigns-research/maternal-request-caesarean/> [Last accessed 15 August 2022].

75% of midwives reporting that current levels of understaffing were 'unsafe': Royal College of Midwives. 2020. *Fears for maternity as staffing shortages hit safety and morale says RCM.* [online] Available at: <https://www.rcm.org.uk/media-releases/2020/november /fears-for-maternity-as-staffing-shortages-hit-safety-and-morale-says-rcm/> [Last accessed 15 August 2022].

one in three doctors working in obstetrics suffer from workplace burnout: Tommy's. 2019. *New mothers and their babies are being put at risk because medics are so exhausted, study warns.* [online] Available at: <https://www.tommys.org/about-us/ charity-news/new-mothers-and-their-babies-are-being-put-risk-because-medics-are -so-exhausted-study-warns> [Last accessed 15 August 2022].

Leah Hazard is an NHS midwife and author of *Hard Pushed: A Midwife's Story*, in which she speaks candidly: Hazard, L., 2019. *Hard Pushed: A Midwife's Story*. London: Arrow Books.

Black women like her were five times more likely than white women to die in pregnancy and childbirth: Knight, M., Bunch, K., Tuffnell, D., Patel, R., Shakespeare, J., Kotnis, R., Kenyon, S., Kurinczuk, J.J. (Eds.) on behalf of MBRRACE-UK. Saving Lives, Improving Mothers' Care – Lessons learned to inform maternity care from the UK and Ireland Confidential Enquiries into Maternal Deaths and Morbidity 2016-18. Oxford: National Perinatal Epidemiology Unit, University of Oxford 2020.

Black women remain four times more likely to die than their white counterparts: Knight, M., Bunch, K., Tuffnell, D., Patel, R., Shakespeare, J., Kotnis, R., Kenyon, S., Kurinczuk, J.J. (Eds.) on behalf of MBRRACE-UK. Saving Lives, Improving Mothers' Care – Lessons learned to inform maternity care from the UK and Ireland Confidential Enquiries into Maternal Deaths and Morbidity 2017-19. Oxford: National Perinatal Epidemiology Unit, University of Oxford 2021.

Black, Asian and ethnic minority women reported feeling humiliated, unsafe and manipulated during labour, as well as being dismissed as 'aggressive':

Black mothers only account for 4% of births in the UK yet are [four] times more likely to die: Office for National Statistics. 2021. *Births and infant mortality by ethnicity, England and Wales*. [online] Available at: <https://www.ons.gov.uk/peoplepopulationand community/healthandsocialcare/childhealth/datasets/birthsandinfantmortalitybyethni cityenglandandwales> [Accessed 15 August 2022].

90% experience some kind of perineal tear, graze or cut (episiotomy: Royal College of Obstetricians and Gynaecologists. *Perineal tears during childbirth*. [online] Available at: <https://www.rcog.org.uk/for-the-public/perineal-tears-and-episiotomies-in -childbirth/perineal-tears-during-childbirth/> [Last accessed 15 August 2022].

at least one in three affected by urinary incontinence: Davies, S., 2014. *The Health of the 51%: Women*. Annual Report of the Chief Medical Officer. [online] Gov.uk. Available at: <https://assets.publishing.service.gov.uk/government/uploads/system/uploads/ attachment_data/file/595439/CMO_annual_report_2014.pdf> [Accessed 15 August 2022].

at 12 and 20 years postnatally, almost a third will have symptoms of pelvic organ prolapse: The British Society of Urogynaecology, 2020. *Injury to Women in Childbirth: The Consequences of Maternal Birth Trauma – written evidence submission*.

Luce Brett, author of *PMSL: Or How I Literally Pissed Myself Laughing and Survived the Last Taboo to Tell the Tale*, writes movingly and candidly about her experiences with postnatal urinary incontinence: Brett, L., 2021. *PMSL: Or How I Literally Pissed Myself Laughing and Survived the Last Taboo to Tell the Tale*. Green Tree.

mothers suffering from incontinence are almost twice as likely to develop postnatal depression: Sword, W., Kurtz Landy, C., Thabane, L., Watt, S., Krueger, P., Farine, D. and Foster, G., 2011. Is mode of delivery associated with postpartum depression at 6 weeks: a prospective cohort study. *BJOG: An International Journal of Obstetrics & Gynaecology*, 118(8), pp.966-977.

91% of respondents saying they weren't given enough advice during pregnancy about postnatal recovery...: Moss, R., 2021. *'I Had No Idea': Women Need To Know What Happens To Their Bodies After Birth*. [online] HuffPost UK. Available at: <https://www .huffingtonpost.co.uk/entry/post-partum-health-mother-and-child_uk_60b0e703e4b 06da8bd75d18a> [Last accessed 15 August 2022].

Brighton and Sussex Hospitals Trust was at the receiving end of a backlash: Baska, M., 2021. *UK's first trans-inclusive birthing language guidelines launch at Brighton hospital. It doesn't tell midwives to stop saying 'mothers'*. [online] Pink News. Available at: <https://www.pinknews.co.uk/2021/02/10/chestfeeding-brighton-sussex-nhs-trust -trans-non-binary-birthing-language-guidelines/> [Last accessed 15 August 2022].

54 trans people gave birth in England between 2016 and 2020, compared to just two between 1996 and 2000: Pearce, R., 2022. *Trans inequalities in English perinatal care*. [online] Dr Ruth Pearce. Available at: <https://ruthpearce.net/2021/09/02/trans -inequalities-in-english-perinatal-care/> [Last accessed 15 August 2022].

Black mothers are more likely than white mothers to experience postnatal depression or anxiety: Watson, H., Harrop, D., Walton, E., Young, A. and Soltani, H., 2019. A systematic review of ethnic minority women's experiences of perinatal mental health conditions and services in Europe. *PLOS ONE*, 14(1), p.e0210587.

...but much less likely to receive treatment: Kozhimannil, K., Trinacty, C., Busch, A., Huskamp, H. and Adams, A., 2011. Racial and Ethnic Disparities in Postpartum Depression Care Among Low-Income Women. *Psychiatric Services*, 62(6), pp.619-625.

half of new mums experience mental health difficulties during pregnancy or within the first year after birth: National Childbirth Trust. 2017. *Nearly half of new mothers with mental health problems don't get diagnosed or treated*. [online] Available at: <https:// www.nct.org.uk/about-us/media/news/nearly-half-new-mothers-mental-health -problems-dont-get-diagnosed-or-treated> [Last accessed 15 August 2022].

one in four new mothers are not asked about their mental health at their six-week check, with 85% saying the appointment focused mainly or equally on the baby's health:

National Childbirth Trust. 2021. *NCT finds a quarter of new mothers are not asked about their mental health.* [online] Available at: <https://www.nct.org.uk/about-us /media/news/nct-finds-quarter-new-mothers-are-not-asked-about-their-mental -health> [Last accessed 15 August 2022].

9. 'DEATH MEANS WE BELIEVE YOU NOW': NEUROTIC MOTHERS IN HEALTHCARE

21-year-old Merryn Crofts became the second person in the UK to have her death officially attributed to severe ME: BBC News. 2018. *'Vindication' for woman who wanted ME on death certificate.* [online] Available at: <https://www.bbc.co.uk/news/ health-44969741> [Last accessed 15 August 2022].

cases like the death of Baby P: McNicoll, A., 2017. *Baby P 10 years on: social work's story.* [online] Community Care. Available at: <https://www.communitycare.co.uk/2017/08 /03/ten-years-baby-p-social-works-story/> [Accessed 15 August 2022].

Steph Nimmo is the author of *Anything For My Child*:

10. 'MENOPAUSAL CRONES': WHEN SEXISM AND AGEISM COLLIDE

just 36% of the 250 respondents felt 'moderately or very prepared' for menopause…: Female Founders Fund. 2020. *Suffering in Silence: The Biases and Data Gaps of Menopause.* [online] Available at: <https://blog.femalefoundersfund.com/suffering-in-silence-the -biases-and-data-gaps-of-menopause-e5f131b4b581> [Last accessed 16 August 2022].

one in four women experiencing menopause symptoms were 'concerned about their ability to cope with life…: Nuffield Health. 2014. *1 in 4 with menopause symptoms worry about coping.* [online] Available at: <https://www.nuffieldhealth.com/article/one-in -four-with-menopause-symptoms-concerned-about-ability-to-cope-with-life> [Last accessed 16 August 2022].

one in five women in perimenopause reduce their hours or don't go for promotions…: Balance. 2021. *Menopause symptoms are killing women's careers, major survey reveals.* [online] Available at: <https://www.balance-menopause.com/news/menopause-symptoms -are-killing-womens-careers-major-survey-reveals/> [Last accessed 16 August 2022].

Vaginal atrophy, which affects one in three women in menopause: Cagnacci, A., Xholli, A., Sclauzero, M., Venier, M., Palma, F. and Gambacciani, M., 2019. Vaginal atrophy across the menopausal age: results from the ANGEL study. *Climacteric*, 22(1), pp.85-89.

Jane Lewis, author of *Me & My Menopausal Vagina*: Lewis, J., 2018. *Me & My Menopausal Vagina.* PAL Books.

65% of women aged 40 and over believe being menopausal has impacted their marriage: Oppenheim, M., 2021. *Almost half of women say they stopped 'having sex while going through menopause'.* [online] The Independent. Available at: <https://www .independent.co.uk/news/uk/home-news/menopause-divorce-reduced-sex-drive -b1889562.html> [Last accessed 16 August 2022].

Mental health issues affect as many as 90% of women during menopause: Oppenheim, M., 2021. *Nine in 10 menopausal women suffer mental health issues, research suggests.* [online] The Independent. Available at: <https://www.independent.co.uk/ independentpremium/menopausal-women-mental-health-b1864347.html> [Accessed 16 August 2022].

women aged 45-64 have the highest female suicide rate in England and Wales: Office for National Statistics. 2021. *Suicides in England and Wales: 2020 registrations.* [online] Available at: <https://www.ons.gov.uk/peoplepopulationandcommunity/birthsd eathsandmarriages/deaths/bulletins/suicidesintheunitedkingdom/2020registrations #suicide-patterns-by-age> [Accessed 16 August 2022].

7% of menopausal women visit their GP more than 10 times and 44% wait at least a year before receiving adequate help or advice: Newson, L. and Lewis, R., 2021. *Delayed diagnosis and treatment of menopause is wasting NHS appointments and resources.*

[online] Newson Health. Available at: <https://d2931px9t312xa.cloudfront.net/menopausedoctor/files/information/632/BMS%20poster%20Louise%20Newson%202021.pdf> [Last accessed 16 August 2022].

stop having periods naturally between 45 and 55 years of age – with 51 the average: NHS Inform. *Menopause.* [online] Available at: <https://www.nhsinform.scot/healthy-living/womens-health/later-years-around-50-years-and-over/menopause-and-post-menopause-health/menopause> [Last accessed 16 August 2022].

POI, which affects around 1% of women under 40: The Daisy Network. *What is POI.* [online] Available at: <https://www.daisynetwork.org/about-poi/what-is-poi/> [Last accessed 16 August 2022].

48%... left with no option but to seek private menopause care, with some of them going thousands of pounds into debt: Oppenheim, M., 2021. *Almost half of menopausal women say they were forced to 'seek private care'.* [online] The Independent. Available at: <https://www.independent.co.uk/news/health/menopause-women-private-healthcare-b1868051.html> [Last accessed 16 August 2022].

menopausal women from ethnic minority communities are more likely than white women to leave the workforce: Women and Equalities Committee, 2022. *Menopause and the workplace.* [online] Available at: <https://publications.parliament.uk/pa/cm5803/cmselect/cmwomeq/91/report.html> [Accessed 16 August 2022].

these patient groups have a higher risk of heart disease: British Heart Foundation. 2021. *How your ethnic background affects your risk of heart and circulatory diseases.* [online] Available at: <https://www.bhf.org.uk/what-we-do/our-research/research-successes/ethnicity-and-heart-disease> [Last accessed 16 August 2022].

Black women are more likely to start menopause up to two years earlier than their white counterparts: El Khoudary, S., Greendale, G., Crawford, S., Avis, N., Brooks, M., Thurston, R., Karvonen-Gutierrez, C., Waetjen, L. and Matthews, K., 2019. The menopause transition and women's health at midlife: a progress report from the Study of Women's Health Across the Nation (SWAN). *Menopause*, 26(10), pp.1213-1227.

Women, for example, outnumber men two to one when it comes to dementia diagnoses: Kiely, A., 2018. *Why is dementia different for women?* [online] Alzheimer's Society. Available at: <https://www.alzheimers.org.uk/blog/why-dementia-different-women> [Last accessed 16 August 2022].

they are more likely to have a lasting impact on low-income women of colour: Tingley, K., 2021. *We Need to Know How Menopause Changes Women's Brains.* [online] The New York Times Magazine. Available at: <https://www.nytimes.com/2021/07/21/magazine/menopause-brains.html> [Last accessed 16 August 2022].

Other possible factors in the dementia gap include sleep disturbances: Mielke, M., Aggarwal, N., Vila-Castelar, C., Agarwal, P., Arenaza-Urquijo, E., Brett, B., Brugulat-Serrat, A., DuBose, L., Eikelboom, W., Flatt, J., Foldi, N., Franzen, S., Gilsanz, P., Li, W., McManus, A., van Lent, D., Milani, S., Shaaban, C., Stites, S., Sundermann, E., Suryadevara, V., Trani, J., Turner, A., Vonk, J., Quiroz, Y. and Babulal, G., 2022. Consideration of sex and gender in Alzheimer's disease and related disorders from a global perspective. *Alzheimer's & Dementia.*

Sociocultural factors like social isolation, and the ability to mask early symptoms through strong verbal skills: Nebel, R., Aggarwal, N., Barnes, L., Gallagher, A., Goldstein, J., Kantarci, K., Mallampalli, M., Mormino, E., Scott, L., Yu, W., Maki, P. and Mielke, M., 2018. Understanding the impact of sex and gender in Alzheimer's disease: A call to action. *Alzheimer's & Dementia*, 14(9), pp.1171-1183.

women with dementia receive less medical attention than men: Cooper, C., Lodwick, R., Walters, K., Raine, R., Manthorpe, J., Iliffe, S. and Petersen, I., 2016. Inequalities in receipt of mental and physical healthcare in people with dementia in the UK. *Age and Ageing.*

declining oestrogen at menopause increases the risk of cardiovascular disease: British Heart Foundation. *Menopause and heart disease.* [online] Available at: <https://www.bhf.org.uk/informationsupport/support/women-with-a-heart-condition/menopause-and-heart-disease> [Last accessed 16 August 2022].

and decreases bone density, putting post-menopausal women and AFAB people at increased risk of osteoporosis: Ji, M. and Yu, Q., 2015. Primary osteoporosis in postmenopausal women. *Chronic Diseases and Translational Medicine*, 1(1), pp.9-13.

An estimated one in two women (compared to one in five men) over 50 will break a bone as a result of osteoporosis: Age UK. *Osteoporosis*. [online] Available at: <https://www.ageuk.org.uk/information-advice/health-wellbeing/conditions-illnesses/osteoporosis/> [Last accessed 16 August 2022].

risk of falling worsens with age: Gale, C., Cooper, C. and Aihie Sayer, A., 2016. Prevalence and risk factors for falls in older men and women: The English Longitudinal Study of Ageing. *Age and Ageing*, 45(6), pp.789-794.

loss of oestrogen loosens the supporting structures of the pelvic floor, leading to problems like urinary incontinence and pelvic organ prolapse: Pisaneschi, S., Palla, G., Spina, S., Bernacchi, G., Cecchi, E., Di Bello, S., Guevara, M., Campelo, A. and Simoncini, T., 2014. Menopause, Aging, Pelvic Organ Prolapse, and Dysfunction. *ISGE Series*, pp.215-224.

women make up nearly 60% of the unpaid carers in the UK and are more likely than men to be 'sandwich carers': Carers UK. *10 facts about women and caring in the UK on International Women's Day*. [online] Available at: <https://www.carersuk.org/news-and-campaigns/features/10-facts-about-women-and-caring-in-the-uk-on-international-women-s-day> [Last accessed 16 August 2022].

Dr Avrum Bluming's book *Oestrogen Matters* explains that oestrogen is not carcinogenic: Bluming, A. and Tavris, C., 2018. *Oestrogen Matters: Why Taking Hormones in Menopause Can Improve Women's Well-Being and Lengthen Their Lives - Without Raising the Risk of Breast Cancer*. Piatkus.

11. 'CAN I SPEAK TO A REAL DOCTOR?' DISMANTLING A SEXIST MEDICAL MODEL

the number of midwives working in England fell by almost 300 in just two months – the fastest drop in over 20 years: Metro. 2021. *The midwife exodus: 'We just can't give mums and babies the care they need'*. [online] Available at: <https://metro.co.uk/2021/10/07/the-midwife-exodus-we-cant-give-mums-and-babies-the-care-they-need-15381667/> [Last accessed 16 August 2022].

57% of midwives are considering leaving within the next year: Royal College of Midwives. 2020. *Fears for maternity as staffing shortages hit safety and morale says RCM*. [online] Available at: <https://www.rcm.org.uk/media-releases/2020/november/fears-for-maternity-as-staffing-shortages-hit-safety-and-morale-says-rcm/> [Last accessed 15 August 2022].

In my local hospital, short-staffing in recent months has led to an increase in negative birth experiences: Facebook post by Lister Stevenage Maternity Voices Partnership. 2 September 2021. *CURRENT SITUATION*. [online] Available at: <https://www.facebook.com/listermaternityvoices/posts/pfbid034GUabsd8U1uUb9zxub5wB1A5NrN3fkJg7eFoLSdzWRc82Fkf2W5sSQim9U2zt7TBl> [Last accessed 16 August 2022].

every single ambulance service in the country is on the highest level of alert... patients are waiting in ambulances for up to 11 hours: The Guardian. 2021. *A&E crisis leaves patients waiting in ambulances outside hospitals for 11 hours*. [online] Available at: <https://www.theguardian.com/uk-news/2021/oct/16/ae-crisis-leaves-patients-waiting-in-ambulances-outside-hospitals-for-11-hours> [Last accessed 16 August 2022].

Jeremy Hunt pledged to expand the GP workforce by 5000 by 2020... the reality in 2021 is that GP numbers have dropped by nearly 1400 instead: Campbell, D., 2021. *'It is with a heavy heart that I leave' – why the unrelieved pressure is pushing GPs to quit*. [online] The Guardian. Available at: <https://www.theguardian.com/society/2021/oct/14/it-is-with-a-heavy-heart-that-i-leave-why-the-unrelieved-pressure-is-pushing-gps-to-quit> [Last accessed 16 August 2022].

In July 2021 the BMA reported that 37% of doctors had experienced verbal abuse in the past month…: BMA, 2021. *BMA calls for Government action to protect GPs and practice staff after horrific violent attack in Manchester GP surgery.* [online] Available at: <https://www.bma.org.uk/bma-media-centre/bma-calls-for-government-action-to-protect-gps-and-practice-staff-after-horrific-violent-attack-in-manchester-gp-surgery> [Last accessed 16 August 2022].

It found that 77% of the 4000 people surveyed were proud of the NHS…: BBC News. 2021. *NHS sparks pride but one in five go private, survey finds.* [online] Available at: <https://www.bbc.co.uk/news/uk-58517295> [Last accessed 16 August 2022].

It is worth noting, though, that the UK has the largest gender health gap in the G20 and the 12th largest in the world: Winchester, N., 2021. *Women's health outcomes: Is there a gender gap?* [online] House of Lords Library. Available at: <https://lordslibrary.parliament.uk/womens-health-outcomes-is-there-a-gender-gap/> [Last accessed 16 August 2022].

77% of the NHS workforce are women: NHS Digital. 2018. *Narrowing of NHS gender divide but men still the majority in senior roles.* [online] Available at: <https://digital.nhs.uk/news/2018/narrowing-of-nhs-gender-divide-but-men-still-the-majority-in-senior-roles> [Last accessed 16 August 2022].

64% of consultants, for example, are men and almost 60% are white: Ethnicity facts and figures. 2021. *NHS workforce.* [online] Available at: <https://www.ethnicity-facts-figures.service.gov.uk/workforce-and-business/workforce-diversity/nhs-workforce/latest#by-ethnicity-and-grade-medical-staff> [Last accessed 16 August 2022].

more than 90% of female doctors had experienced sexism at work in the past two years: British Medical Association, 2021. *Sexism in medicine.* [online] British Medical Association. Available at: <https://www.bma.org.uk/media/4487/sexism-in-medicine-bma-report.pdf> [Last accessed 16 August 2022].

the 2020 survey of all (clinical and non-clinical) NHS staff found that, in the previous 12 months, 17% of ethnic minority staff, 12% of gay or lesbian staff and 13% of bisexual staff had experienced discrimination: NHS, 2020. *Staff Survey 2020.* [online] Available at: <https://www.nhsstaffsurveys.com/>.

A 2021 BMA survey found that nearly 80% of doctors have experienced 'moral distress': British Medical Association, 2021. *Moral distress and moral injury: Recognising and tackling it for UK doctors.* [online] British Medical Association. Available at: <https://www.bma.org.uk/media/4209/bma-moral-distress-injury-survey-report-june-2021.pdf> [Last accessed 16 August 2022].

there were more than 93,000 full-time equivalent vacancies across the NHS in June 2021: NHS Digital. 2021. *NHS Vacancy Statistics England April 2015 – June 2021 Experimental Statistics.* [online] Available at: <https://digital.nhs.uk/data-and-information/publications/statistical/nhs-vacancies-survey/april-2015---june-2021-experimental-statistics> [Last accessed 16 August 2022].

84% of respondents reported feeling that they had not been listened to by healthcare staff: Department of Health & Social Care, 2022. *Women's Health Strategy for England.* [online] Gov.uk. Available at: <https://assets.publishing.service.gov.uk/government/uploads/system/uploads/attachment_data/file/1092439/Women_s-Health-Strategy-England-web.pdf> [Last accessed 16 August 2022].

ACKNOWLEDGEMENTS

Unlike our healthcare system, this book was created by and for women – not just me, but all those women who inspired it. Their experiences, insights and wisdom are *Rebel Bodies'* heart and soul, and it quite simply would not exist without the 100+ women whose voices fill these pages. I'm also grateful to the smaller number of men and non-binary people who shared their own important perspectives, whether as patients or healthcare professionals. Thank you to each and every one of you for speaking out and trusting me to tell your stories. Particular thanks go to Philippa Willitts, Athena Lamnisos, Dr Alison Berner and Dr Ben Vincent for their early reading and expert feedback.

Thanks also to the Hysterical Women community – everyone who's written for, engaged with and shared the blog, and provided moral or financial support along the way. I have learned, and continue to learn, so much from you. Likewise, to the writers and editors I've had the privilege of working with, learning from, and being challenged by over the last decade; I know I'm a better journalist because of you.

I am so thankful for the endless cheerleading of my agent, Julia Silk, who always just gets it. Finding her really was a little lockdown love story. Thank you, Julia, for believing in me and this book, for always being on the other end of the phone to put the world to rights with me, and for your wisdom and guidance on everything from publishing to childbirth.

Thank you to Charlotte, Holly, both Sarahs, Katherine and the wider team at Bloomsbury for your flexibility, vision and all your hard work in bringing my book to life. It's been such a joy and an honour to publish with you.

To Sam Couchman, Roisin McLaughlin-Dowd, Hannah Robinson-Pickett, Paul and Rachael Graham, and my work wife Philippa Willitts (again!): thank you for being such wonderful friends and sounding boards, particularly over the last two years. For brainstorming with me, celebrating with me, endlessly bigging up my work to other people, and always challenging my self-doubt.

Thanks to my parents for their love, support, and instilling a lifelong belief in the power of words. More recently, special thanks to my mum for all the unpaid childcare, the 24/7 WhatsApp parenting support service, and generally preserving my sanity through all the challenges of simultaneously bringing a baby and a book into the world.

Above all I am endlessly grateful to Josh – for absolutely everything, but especially for all the tea, two-course toast and cuddles that fuelled long days of writing and editing. None of it could have happened without your constant, unwavering love, support and domestic labour. And finally, my son – this book's twin – who has made this last year the most wonderful rollercoaster of my life.

INDEX